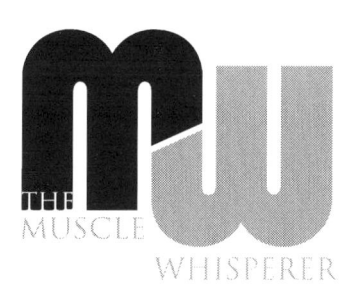

THE MUSCLE WHISPERER

THE KEYS TO UNLOCKING YOUR BACK PAIN

SOPHIA KUPSE

For more information please visit: **www.themusclewhisperer.co.uk**

THE MUSCLE WHISPERER
THE KEYS TO UNLOCKING BACK PAIN

Copyright © 2014
The Muscle Whisperer - The Keys to Unlocking your Back Pain
By Sophia Kupse

Published in the UK 2014 by Sophia Kupse.

All rights reserved. No part of this publication may be represented, stored in or introduced into a retrieval system or transmitted in any form or by any means (electronic, mechanical, photocopying, recording or otherwise) without the prior written permission of the publisher.

This book is sold subject to the condition that it shall not, by way of trade or otherwise, be lent, resold, hired out or otherwise circulated without the publisher's consent in any form of binding or cover other than that in which it is published and without a similar condition including this condition being imposed on the subsequent purchaser.

This book contains advise and information relating to health care. It is not intended to replace medical advise and should be used in supplement to regular care by your doctor. The publisher and author relinquish liability for any medical outcomes that may occur as a result of applying the methods suggested in this book.

Printed in the UK by CreateSpace.

ISBN-13: 978-1492713142
ISBN-10: 1492713147

DEDICATION

I dedicate this book to my loving family; my mother who taught me how to survive against the odds, work through every challenge and gave me the wisdom of her inspirational words. My sister Val & husband Greg, who have been my rock and proof readers, putting their precious time together to one side, whilst putting my needs first. My brother John for all his technical expertise, saving my work before I lost it all, in order to get the book published. To my two beautiful children Laura & Alex, who have been my greatest teachers on the journey of self discovery.

I would also like to thank all my clients who over the years have made the 'Langellotti Tri-Therapy' evolve into the most revolutionary advanced holistic back pain treatment on the market today. It's been a privilege helping you all overcome your pain and a pleasure knowing you have become stronger because of it.

To Katherine
with love
Anne x

CONTENTS

	Acknowledgments	6
	Introduction	7
Chapter 1	HOW I GOT HERE	14
Chapter 2	UNDERSTANDING BACK PAIN	25
Chapter 3	FACT VERSUS FICTION	33
Chapter 4	THE BRAIN	42
Chapter 5	FEEDING OUR MUSCLES	55
Chapter 6	EXERCISE- DO YOU OR DON'T YOU	68
Chapter 7	TAKE CONTROL	82
Chapter 8	THE KEYS TO UNLOCKING YOUR BACK PAIN	92
	Final Word	*106*
	References	*99*

ACKNOWLEDGMENTS

TO ANTHONY ROBBINS, LIFE COACH & AUTHOR - who transformed my limiting beliefs from his amazing Cardiff Fire Walk Event in 1999 & his bestselling book 'Awaken the Giant Within.' He truly was the catalyst that started a sequence of change that helped transform me, to create the successful person I am today. His work continues to motivate & inspire me.

TO NEIL BOOTH, WEB DESIGNER & AUTHOR - for always believing in me and my brand, developing my website **www.themusclewhisperer.co.uk** for all to share. Your love and passion shows through your work and I am truly blessed to have you as a friend.

TO JANEY LEE GRACE, HOLISTIC LIVING EXPERT & AUTHOR - for inspiring me to write my first book, telling me it was my duty to share my knowledge with the world and I did.

TO FIONA KIRK, TOP UK NUTRITIONIST & AUTHOR - who saved me from self publishing disaster.

TO MAX MORRIS, MILKBAR CREATIVE - for making the dream come true.

TO DAVID CLARKE, ROCK PR - for having faith in me and letting the world know.

INTRODUCTION

As a Holistic Practitioner working with Eastern & Western therapies for over 20 years, I was searching for a natural treatment that would help people suffering from any form of neck, shoulder and back pain. My quest was triggered by my own personal experience with lower back pain, here is how it began.

MY STORY

It was Christmas Eve 1987, I was 23 years old and leaving midnight mass. It was a clear, cold, crisp night, with a touch of frost beginning to form on all the cars parked bumper to bumper outside the church. The service was crammed to the door with every sinner seeking inspiration & forgiveness, including me. As I searched for my keys, I looked up at the sky, not a cloud was in sight just beautiful twinkling stars. The quicker I left, the closer I would be to getting home and starting my Christmas holiday with the family. I could see my warm breath cutting through the cold air, rolling off the windscreen like a wave. I clicked my seat belt into place, starting to feel excited by the most wonderful time of the year and I felt truly blessed. I turned the key in the ignition, indicated that I was pulling out and slowly manoeuvred the car onto the busy main road.

I had only gone a few yards and was still in first gear, when I saw a pair of headlights veering towards me. I couldn't understand why they were there, on my side of the road, when they should have been on the opposite side. Everything after that thought, happened in slow motion. I was hit head on at 50 miles an hour whilst practically stationary, by a drunk driver who had had an epileptic fit at the wheel. He had taken his dad's car that night, without permission, despite having had his licence revoked due to his medical condition. As he blacked out, his foot hit the accelerator pedal, heading towards me like a runaway train, completely out of control. I took all the impact, as the speed at which his car hit me, crushed my car and me with it. He received a scratch to the head and walked away from the collision scene, whilst it took a crew of six firemen over an hour to cut me out. Within minutes, the saloon car I was driving had shrunk down to the size of a Mini. I remember to this day how one of the fire officers just kept talking to me in an effort to keep me conscious. I could barely breathe as my face had smashed into the steering wheel which had also compressed my chest (airbags had not yet been invented). I knew that night if I blacked out at any point, I would never wake up in this world again. All I could do was focus on what little breath was coming out of me and pray to the God I had just left, to keep me alive. I knew I had a greater purpose and if given the chance, I would prove it.

During the church service that evening, I had prayed for an old school friend who had recently been killed in a head-on collision only a few weeks before Christmas. As I prayed, I reflected on how this was something I would never want to go through and now, only an hour later, I was fighting for my life for that exact reason. Why was God testing me, surely it was not my time to leave yet? The paramedic treating me with oxygen in the ambulance could not understand how I had remained conscious. My blood pressure had dropped so low, I should have been well and truly under by now. I was blue lighted direct to A&E where I experienced a very different Christmas that year. This was my first long stay in hospital since the age of 5, when I had suffered a bout of gastroenteritis and was imprisoned in a glass cell for a month, labelled 'Infectious diseases'. I was kept under observation like a tropical specimen, constantly monitored by doctors and nurses. My poor mother's face was a distressing picture. Like all mothers, she wore a happy smile trying to console me behind a pane of glass, when really she was crying as much as me. Now as she visited me in hospital on Christmas Day, she had that same look on her face, trying to stretch it into a reassuring smile, when really she wanted to scream. I was all tubed and wired up to breathing monitors and a variety of complex apparatus to control my body's functions. My face was distorted beyond recognition, which was everyone's concern. Would I ever look like me again? I never looked in a mirror for the first six weeks of my recovery.

In the early stages of my rehabilitation programme, doctors were already deciding whether I would be spending the rest of my life in a wheelchair, but I had other ideas. Recovering from a punctured lung, cracked ribs, a damaged sciatic nerve, broken nose and jaw, severe bruising from head to toe, these were just a small selection of the less problematic issues I was challenged with. I felt I had become old before my time. Countless visits to the hospital, physiotherapist and osteopath helped, but could not resolve the damage that had now become a part of me. It was at this point during my convalescence I discovered that if I wanted my old life back, and a future having a family, I would have to change my approach and master a new plan. Determination, drive, passion and the will to succeed had to be my motivation and failure was never an option. I had to train my thoughts in order to bring about mental, as well as physical change. I had to battle with my beliefs to convince my body that I was now fully recovered and back to being my former self. When you think like this, you have to believe it as if the change has already happened and it is your reality. There is no room for doubt or pretending it's not happened: in order to move a mountain you have to become part of it. As they say in Yorkshire, 'Where there's a will, there's a way.'

I had read many books about the power of the mind and how the mind cannot distinguish the difference between reality and fantasy. I was extremely thankful for my obsession with the written word from an early age, which started the moment I read my first Janet & John book. Books gave me the power to escape into my deepest thoughts and release the most amazing world of fantasy. I had a great appetite for fiction, such as Enid Blyton's Famous Five, The Malory Towers series and in my later teens, Harold Robbins & Jackie Collins! I lived out those stories in my daydreams, so you can see, I had a very vivid imagination which paid dividends in aiding my recovery. Before starting the experiment, I had to introduce a few key ingredients in order for my mind to accept my thoughts as reality. I created a visual storyboard, with pictures of destinations I would travel to, walks I would participate in, cars I would drive, the home of my dreams and the family and friends who would be sharing it with me. I had strength of mind, the willpower to succeed and a clear goal: to be pain free and fully mobile again. I had read many medical books that advocated mind over matter and highlighted successful case studies to illustrate how having a positive mindset and focusing on the outcome, you can change anything. Remember, this was the mid 1980's before books like 'The Secret' had been written. I suppose I was ahead of my time when it came to believing in dreams and making the impossible possible.

This was my test, my experiment on me. If I failed, I had nothing to lose as I couldn't make myself any worse than I was, and I had time on my hands to do it. So instead of focusing on the negative and re-living what I had been through, I started to practice a primitive version of meditation. I found that by tapping into the power of my subconscious mind, I could control my thought patterns and any feelings of pain, allowing my body's natural self-healing system to take over and speed up recovery. Wanting to get better, mentally and physically was key to the success of my recovery. If I had wallowed in my past and pressed the repeat button on the accident, then every time I spoke to someone about it, I would be re-living that moment again, and my life would revolve around that incident, creating my own 'groundhog day.' I would never make any further progress because I would be living in the past, putting my present and future on hold.

How many people do you know (or are you one of them) that live in the past, that blames your lack of progress on a bad relationship, a stale job, financial over-commitment or an illness you couldn't get over. By constantly talking about it, you have become the victim of it not the survivor, which is what I wanted to be. It's what you have to be in order to move forward in your life. The emotional stress you hold onto starts to manifest in your body and is held in our back muscles, until one day you feel it as physical pain.

Day after day I focused on seeing myself growing stronger. When any pain arose, I would sit and clear my thoughts. I focused on my breath and controlled any feelings that I felt throughout my body. I felt it get less and less, until it was no longer there. How powerful that exercise was! I hated taking tablets especially painkillers, so this was my nirvana, I had reached a place in my mind that gave me the freedom to control my pain. It takes a lot of focus, concentration and self belief to achieve this and for many people, it will seem an almost impossible task. For me, I had achieved the solution to controlling my pain and with that came mobility and freedom to live my life the way I wanted it to be, the way I had imagined.

CONCLUSION

Even though I had long term scar tissue created from the injuries I sustained from the accident, I made a full recovery over nine months to the amazement of the medics. I had at least prevented the doctor's prediction of life in a wheelchair. I knew as I got older, that my body would start to breakdown and take a lot longer to recover, so managing any pain would be an ongoing practice. I learned that every time I got angry or had to deal with a stressful situation, my back pain would trigger, yet every time I was happy, having fun or relaxed, no pain would occur. Additional research later would lead me to understand why. That Christmas Eve night, I now believe, was the night I received the best gift of all and at the same time faced my biggest fears. The accident triggered my journey into a new vocation that would see me helping hundreds of people around the world for the rest of my life.

I began training in holistic therapies and learnt over seven disciplines of massage. My knowledge on anatomy & physiology grew and I built a successful back pain clinic where I lived. I continued to study, as I craved to understand more facts about how the mind affects the body. This helped me make a clear connection between the two, proving that emotional stress, more than physical stress, has an immediate impact in creating back pain. Studying 'La Stone Therapy' back in 1997 taught me the positive effects of heat and ice application to the body. I was fascinated at the speed in which it worked; activating the body's natural healing process, leaving the client feeling calm after a physical treatment. Like a scientist in pursuit of a breakthrough antidote or a chef searching for the ultimate accolade, a Michelin star, I was exploring the best methods that combined to make the ultimate synergistic back pain treatment. It had to deliver fast results with no trauma to the muscle or patient. I began blending together a variety of massage techniques, essential oils and the two natural elements of volcanic heat and ice marble to form what has now become known as 'LT Therapy.' I had discovered the perfect recipe for muscle recovery, eliminating back pain caused by emotional and physical stress. All three elements had to be used in order to achieve successful results, so the 'Tri-Method system' was born. Had I found the key to unlocking the door to muscular back pain and bringing about a revolutionary change in the way we treat it?

This book was written to help people understand why back pain has rapidly grown worldwide to become the silent epidemic. I show how you can quickly recover using proven techniques that work. The book includes real case studies of actual clients I have treated; only their names have been changed to protect their identity. I hope that when you finish reading the book, you will have a better understanding of back pain and how to use all or some of the proven methods to heal your back for life.

1
HOW I GOT HERE

My journey has not been an easy one, on the road to developing my skills and abilities to do my specialised work. I believe that our life challenges are an opportunity for us to grow and enrich who we are, no matter how dark those moments can be. I have been to places and experienced great depths of sadness, loss and pain which started from the tender age of five. Each decade of my life, from birth to my 50th year, has been filled with these challenges, lessons of life which I have used to develop all my abilities.

Many would say that I was robbed of my childhood and had to grow up before my time, but I see those very dark days as a time where my strongest roots were formed, that created the foundations of the person I am today. I always laugh when journalists who interview me (or anyone for that matter) ask the question 'Do you have any regrets?' 'Of course I don't' is my answer, as to have regrets about any of your experiences means you haven't learned the purpose of what it was about. If you regret anything that was in your life, no matter how distressing, then you have already created a paradox. You've challenged, or questioned a past decision, placing doubt on your actions taken. This in turn creates guilt, which leads to pain, which is negative and toxic, poisoning our 'whole' self, mind, body & spirit. So many of us carry those lifetime regrets inside of us, like an invisible cross strapped to our chest or a huge backpack the size of something you would carry on a 365 day world expedition. The weight of such a burden is too much for a person and the overspill is physical pain in the body. In Western medicine our back, the trunk, carries some of the major and biggest muscle groups of the body, where physical stress impacts. In Eastern holistic medicine, the back represents our past, our life's history, where our emotional stress is held; is it any wonder why so many of us are suffering from back pain? We are a society that has always been led to believe that any neck, shoulder and back pain is associated with a physical trauma or action, which is not always the case.

I believe I had to go through almost half a century of challenges in order to become the person I am today, 'The Muscle Whisperer;' an interpreter of muscular pain, a back reader, a translator of muscle language. By living through decades of challenges, I have developed a greater understanding of living in today's fanatical lifestyle, allowing me to empathise with people's circumstances, whether they have had financial difficulties, pressure at work, health issues or struggled with relationships, as I have had to face all those issues myself. I have become deeply intuitive, raising my awareness to a level that enables me to tune myself in to the client's aura or electrical energy field. As a holistic practitioner, it is my job to be able to relate to the person I am treating in order for me to achieve a successful result. When my client gives me permission to work on their back, they are asking me to take away their pain, releasing them from a lifetime of suffering. I see this as a gift and it gives me great pleasure to ensure that by the time their treatment has ended, they feel a weight has truly been lifted from their shoulders.

So can I really make such a bold statement and say that 'we can enjoy a life without back pain'? Well I'm here to prove that we can. As a former back pain sufferer, I made it my personal mission to eliminate my own back pain and help show others how to do the same with theirs. By creating four key changes we can unlock back pain forever, but in order to sustain it for life, it has to be practiced daily. My treatment is not for everyone, only those who are ready and willing to let go of the emotional and physical pain trapped in their neck, shoulder & back muscles. When they are released, a great sense of freedom, lightness and flexibility can be felt. In order to maintain that state, you need to practice the four keys daily. Are you ready to make that change? I have treated hundreds of clients over the past 20 years suffering from all forms of back pain and those few that do make those daily changes, have remained pain-free for life. It takes a lot of work and commitment, but like anything, once you have mastered it, it will become your natural way of life.

WHY 'THE MUSCLE WHISPERER'?

During my years in clinic, I noticed that over 85% of people I treated had never suffered any form of physical trauma or accident leading to their back pain. They had started with back pain for no apparent reason and tried to justify their pain by linking it to a small physical task they had recently carried out, like lifting a box or getting out of bed awkwardly. I wanted to find out why there were such a high number of these cases and if there were any common factors linking them together. I went back over two decades and reviewed all my cases. I knew I would find something, and I did. I discovered that the physical symptoms of back pain are only a secondary effect, originating from and caused by the persons emotional state and 21st century stress. Bingo! This was the link, the common factor that connected my cases together-STRESS. I referenced the holistic methods of eastern medicine, which uses the balance of 'Yin & Yang' as an important feature of wellbeing in the body. They refer to the left side of the body as male energy and the right side of the body as female energy. For total wellbeing this balance must always be maintained or over a long period of time dis-ease takes place.

When we bring two great worlds of holistic medicine together, we see that western medicine shows us that muscles have muscle memory and in eastern medicine, the back represents our past history. Like a timeline, the base represents the foundations of our life, (from childhood) and the upper back relates to our current situation. When the back harbours pain due to a build-up of pressure and knots, the balance of 'Yin & Yang' is out of sync. Treating the sufferer as a 'whole' person means treating their emotional, physical and spiritual state, as in eastern medicine, whereas western medicine just treats the symptom.

As the founder of one of the most advanced holistic back pain treatments on the market today, the 'Langellotti Tri-Therapy' (LT Therapy as it is generally known), I incorporated the best of both eastern and western holistic medicine, in order to bring about an amazing level of change to mind, body and spirit, restoring balance and eliminating back pain for life. My 'Tri-Therapy' method is a three-way treatment using my advanced massage technique, volcanic heat and ice marble. My stones have been with me for the past 16 years and when I use them, they are an extension of my hands. They are not there as a labour saving device or to save my hands, but rather to assist in the recovery of the muscle. They each have a specific role to play. The volcanic stones were formed from a South American Volcano and tumbled a thousand times to reach their smooth state. Only volcanic stone can be used as it retains heat for a longer period of time, a key part in the recovery of the muscle. Set at 62 degrees, I use the heat to detox the muscle and the client instantly feels pain diminishing. The gentle yet powerful action of this natural element, removes lactic acid build up quickly, de-stressing the muscle. The client feels pain melt away. The white marble was sourced from Carerra in Tuscany, Italy. Set at zero degrees, it is a natural anti-inflammatory which super charges the muscle by increasing oxygen and nutrients back to the tissue. Flexibility, mobility and balance are instantly restored to the treated area. An intuitive touch, years of experience and a passion to succeed where other methods fail, is the driving force behind the Muscle Whisperer's mission.

My aim is to achieve successful results with every client I treat and in doing so, I am getting nearer to closing the gap on back pain. My clients all leave with a clear understanding that if they want to enjoy a good recovery from back pain for days, weeks, months and even years, like me, they need to adjust the way they deal with the daily pressures of life and introduce some positive changes to getting more balance back. It's all about learning to take control, rather than constantly reacting to life, putting you first in order to help others. 'I thought this was a book about understanding back pain' I hear you shout! Yes it is, but in order to eliminate and control pain, you need to change the way you think and approach it.

People usually come to me as their last resort before going down the route of operations, which can be unsuccessful. I don't claim to be a magician who can eliminate your pain in an instant, but I can offer you a natural, organic solution to dealing with it. In order for you to appreciate the level of my work, you need to understand how I got to be whom I am today – the Muscle Whisperer.

ONCE UPON A TIME...

I was born in Bradford on 8th September 1963 to European parents. My elder brother had arrived 11 months prior to my birthday and then there was my younger brother the following year, who was still-born. My younger sister came exactly six years and a day before my 6th birthday and we were to become lifelong friends. In 1963 England was welcoming the swinging 60's with Beatlemania, the public were coping with The Big Freeze, the Great Train Robbery had baffled the police and

Steve McQueen had just released 'The Great Escape'. People had to live on what they had, there were no extended mortgages, credit cards or easy loan facilities. Cars were seen as a luxury for the rich and no one on our street owned a telephone. Both my parents had arrived in England through hardship; my father left Hungary during the 1956 revolution, waiting for the ship to Florida that never came, so England became his new home and work was found in the textile city of Bradford. My mother, who was orphaned at the age of three, escaped her home town in the province of Caserta near Naples, when the convent she grew up in was forced to close. At the age of 18, she got passage and a contract as a seamstress in Sussex, England. Two years later, she moved to Bradford where the textile mills gave her a fresh start and she met my father.

My mother was always a thrifty person, cleverly saving money by making all our clothes. She could sew, hand stitch, knit, embroider, and make fine lace. We had every season in our wardrobe covered. Her cooking skills were outstanding as she produced not only British dishes that she learnt from her friends in the mills, but her own cuisine as well as my father's Hungarian dishes. By the time my sister came along, I was six and my mum's sous chef. I learnt that chores came before playtime, so I never really got much free time in my younger years, as there were always never ending chores to do sandwiched between school.

I believe my early start in learning how to run a house and cook a variety of continental dishes, as well as squeezing in an education, made me adapt quickly to situations. I became very intuitive and sensitive to other people's needs and my organisational skills were one of my main strengths, ensuring no one ever got missed. My father had an allotment close to the house where he grew flowers, herbs and soft fruits. He would make jams for the winter with the summer fruits and dry herbs to use in cooking all year round. He was also a part time herbalist, like his mother and great grandmother. He would make lots of natural remedies and whenever we fell or had a cold, my Dad would be there making a poultice from nettles, or cream from calendula flowers to heal our cuts and grazes. I believe most of my natural ability to work intuitively in the field of holistic medicine came from him and although he has passed away, I feel a part of him always with me, looking over my shoulder influencing my thoughts when deciding on which essential oils to use. My mother went on to train as a nurse and worked with young disabled patients who had Multiple Sclerosis as well as TB, which was rife in Bradford in the 1970's. It was her work as a nurse and the lack of an automated lifting system which had not yet been developed, that caused her back problems in later years. Despite being only 5ft tall she was extremely strong, slim and petite, a lot like me, but was considering early retirement due to the pain which started to travel down her legs. My mother became my first client to benefit from 'LT Therapy', on whom I successfully achieved great results from such primitive beginnings. I named my treatment 'Langellotti' after her (and my) Italian heritage. This is her story...

MARIA'S STORY

Maria's lower back pain started half way through her nursing career, she was 42 years old. She had had a hysterectomy at the age of 37 and was beginning to suspect that her lower back muscles had become weak from the surgery, as the muscles were all interlinked, causing her sciatica. When I started to work on her back, I knew my mother's history, how she was orphaned at the age of three, brought up by very strict nuns and never allowed to express her creative side. She married my father in 1961 and by 1962 my brother was born, quickly followed by me in 1963 and then another pregnancy in 1964. The third baby, our brother, was stillborn and my mother blamed her quick, successive pregnancies, poor diet and lack of vitamins due to poverty, as the main cause of his death. In reality this was never the case, but she took on the need to carry this lifelong responsibility nevertheless.

She was extremely successful at whatever she tried her hand at and had an exceptional palate when it came to rustic cooking. Glamorous dinner parties were held at our home, when friends flocked to taste her cuisine. It was one of the few ways my mother learnt how to express her creative side, as well as dressmaking. I became her little chef and learnt that in order to create a successful dish, you had to keep tasting the food, in order to bring out the beautiful flavours of the meal. I don't think at the time I really appreciated what I was doing, and how my love of cooking and baking would ignite the passion inside me that eventually would be a key emotion in my future work.

In order to release her lower back pain, I had to work on her neck and shoulders to discharge the toxic build up of lactic acid held in the muscles. When too much adrenaline and cortisol is produced they crystallise, forming pockets of knots which restrict blood flow and cause pressure to build in that area. Adrenaline pumps out whenever we get too stressed; the body recognises that we need the extra 'fight or flight' response in our system and boom! It's there. Maria had lived almost a lifetime in the 'fight or flight' response mode and it was beginning to show in her back. The main area of concern was her left side, which in eastern medicine reflects male energy (see Fig 1). I knew of the guilt she carried regarding my younger brother's death and how difficult a man my father was to live with; for all the good qualities he had, there were equally, many bad. He had mentally and physically bullied her throughout their marriage and with the loss of her parents as a child, she had very low self esteem. She was a very loyal and trustworthy person, but my father had suffered with many years of chronic depression which went undiagnosed and caused so much unnecessary pain in the family.

I found it a challenge to tell my mother that her main body of pain had come from not only her guilt about the baby, but due to my father's behaviour, especially since he had started having several affairs.

My mother was now 52 years of age and I had been treating her for three months. At first she found it unbelievably difficult to accept my theory as to why she was suffering from her back pain, as she was truly convinced it was 100% down to her physical job. She point blank refused to listen, dismissing it as a nonsense theory, something I developed from my imagination. Sometimes, people cannot face the truth, they would rather live with the fear and guilt they have carried around for so long, making it become their reality. The turning point came when I started to back track her life, highlighting the fact that her pain actually started at 42, coinciding with the exact same time when my father had begun having his affairs. My mother began to realise that she had held on to all her pain and was blaming physical things like her operation, the lifting at work, when really it was down to the guilt she carried for a lost child and the anger she felt about my father's behaviour. She had so many negative emotions that needed to be released in a positive way, but she had to make that decision herself. I never tell my clients what to do, I just advise them to review their lives and take things into their own hands, wherever possible, in order to release their pain and achieve a positive result.

My mother, Maria, finally made peace with herself regarding the death of her stillborn child and made the decision to leave my father whom she divorced in 1987, setting herself free to start a new life, the way she wanted to live it. Her back pain diminished almost overnight as she finally stood up for herself. She continued to work as a nurse until her retirement with no recurring back pain.

CONCLUSION

Maria's story is not an unusual one; when one partner is unfaithful, suffers chronic depression or is a mental/physical bully, the sufferer takes on the responsibility, sheltering the shame of the behaviour of the person they trusted. My mother was no exception, in fact, her beliefs as a Roman Catholic did nothing but make the situation worse, as she believed it was her duty as a wife to stand by her husband, regardless of his abusive behaviour.

Maria is now a spritely 75 year old, living her life to the full. Releasing her back pain over 20 years ago, gave her a second chance to have the life she always dreamed of, a life of freedom. You are only a prisoner when you give in to fear, fear of the unknown. Better to face the challenges that lie ahead and become a stronger person because of them, than to die never knowing what might have been. I learnt so much from treating my mother, I had a deeper understanding of how a poor relationship can cause deep back pain. When you are not in a happy state, your whole body implodes, you walk in a concaved manner with rounded shoulders, and your muscles are tight, holding on to emotions like anger, upset, guilt and disappointment. When you are happy and truly in love with life, you open up like a flower, making a silent statement to everyone 'look at me, I'm really happy'. Your muscles are soft and playful just like your manner. Which state do you prefer to live in?

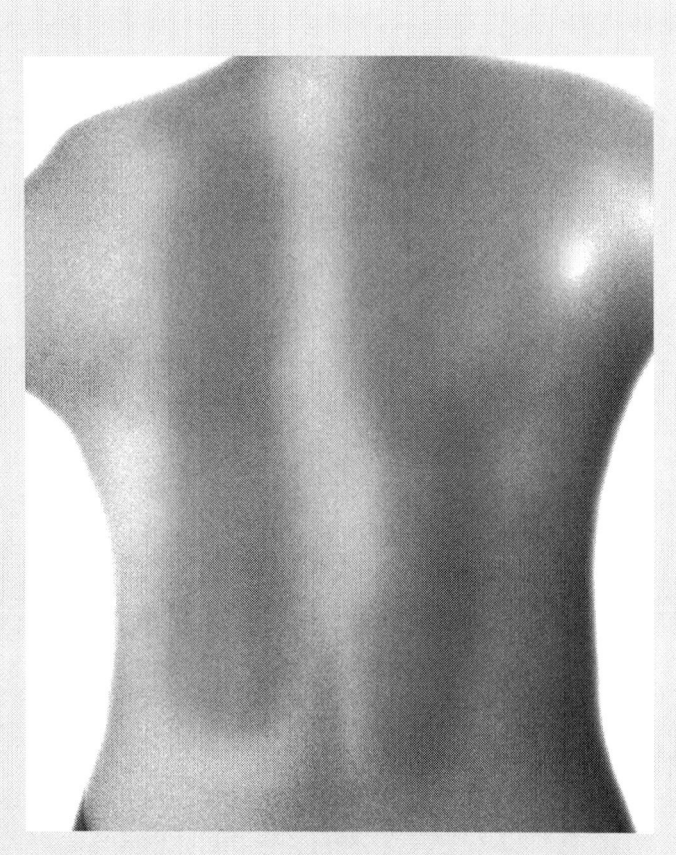

Fig 1 - Photo shows both sides of the back with dark areas, but left side relating to male energy more congested.

24 HOW I GOT HERE

2
UNDERSTANDING BACK PAIN

CHALLENGING THE MYTH

In order to understand back pain we need to consider what causes it. For many people back pain can be triggered by everyday activities at home or at work, or it can develop gradually over time as a result of prolonged sitting or standing or even lifting badly. Classic causes people associate with back pain include:

- Bending awkwardly or for long periods
- Lifting, carrying, pushing or pulling incorrectly
- Slouching in chairs
- Twisting
- Over-stretching
- Driving in a hunched position or driving for long periods without taking a break
- Overuse of the muscles, usually due to sport or repetitive movements
- Sitting at the computer for long periods of time.

Sometimes back pain develops suddenly for no apparent reason. Some people just wake up one morning with back pain and have no idea what has caused it. Now I'm challenging you to think of another reason, one that has not been mentioned, is backed by scientific evidence, but is rarely linked to back pain, answer – stress.

Stress is the new plague of the 21st century. It grows rapidly like a silent epidemic, makes the same impact, creates discomfort and you only know about it when it's gone too far. Many people don't even know the perimeter of where back pain begins and ends, so I'll clarify. When I treat people suffering from back pain, it includes the whole neck, shoulders, mid and lower back, not just the mid to lower back as most people assume. The diagram below shows a simple illustration of our back muscles, so you are always aware of where pain can strike.

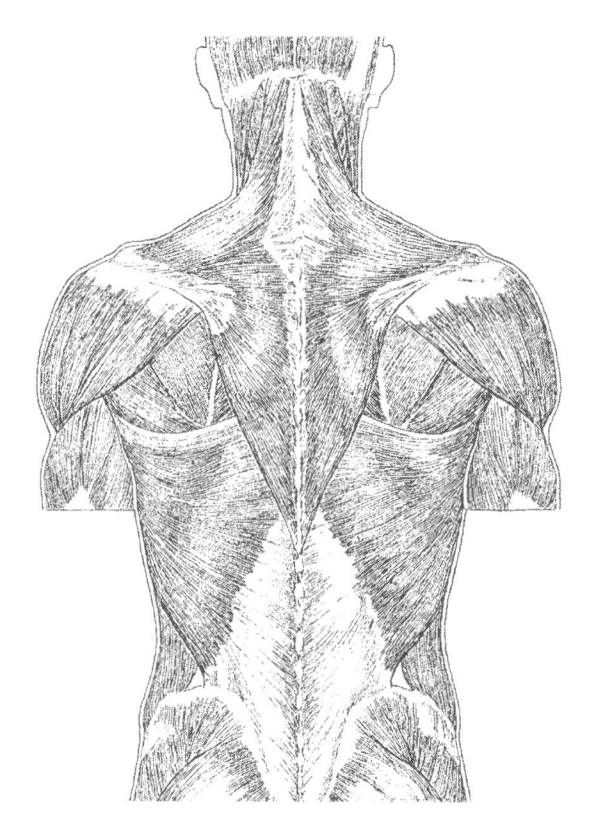

When we look at the human anatomy, the back is the mother ship of our body, housing some of our biggest muscle groups- is it any wonder we feel our pain in those areas? The torso is where the head and neck connect to, as well as the arms and legs. When we start to suffer from back pain, our life is dominated by it. We can't seem to function normally. Our lives are overtaken by the pain and it starts to affect our daily routine; our body begins to move differently to accommodate the pain. We stop doing activities that we loved because of the pain. We actually start to include pain in our conversation with others, suddenly we become the victim, pain is now in control; it has entered our world and found a nice cosy place to live. We have invited this unwelcomed guest; we've set another place at the table and ensured that it will always have a position to feast on.

Soon the pain begins to have a life of its own and spreads to other parts of the body, as we allow our subconscious thoughts to manifest even more. During my years in clinic, I treated hundreds of people who made their mental stress become their physical pain, almost like carrying an invisible crucifix.

It was a symbol of their silent suffering, their spirit reaching out for someone to rescue them from their pain, take away their fears and help them to reset the balance button. Solutions to life's challenges are never that simple. Many people look to me as their Guru, Saviour, and the person who could 'magic' their back pain away, making their lives instantly better. Yes, for a brief moment, I have that effect, but in order to continue experiencing the benefits from my treatment, they have to change the way they tackle daily stress and make adjustments to their lifestyle, or the cycle of back pain will continue. I give them the suit of armour required to safeguard their muscles, but I cannot wear it for them.

Each day we live with new challenges, such as handling the demands of a new job or juggling an existing workload that has been increased with no extra pay. Welcoming a new baby into your life or saying goodbye to a loved one in death. Going through a painful divorce/separation or living with an unresolved family feud or abusive relationship. Caring for family members, especially the elderly, disabled or sick. Discovering deceit, handling shock, the stress list is endless, all adding to the syndrome of back pain.

In an ideal world, the neck, shoulder & back muscles should always be in a soft flexible state, enabling optimum movement with minimal impact to the skeletal structure. If the back muscles become too tight, due to a high level of lactic acid build up, movement is restricted. This in turn puts pressure on the surrounding joints and tendons which starts to impact bone and soft tissue. If the major muscles that support the spine become inflexible, then this limits movement in the surrounding muscles. The higher the impact to the back muscles, the greater the pressure builds against the spine. If the spine no longer moves freely, then this impinges on the performance of the discs. Over time, deterioration will occur and conditions such as prolapsed disc transpire. The number of spinal issues and rotator cuff injuries has risen greatly since the 1980's. Doctors are uncertain why, but a more sedentary lifestyle both at home and work, inactivity, obesity and poor core strength due to fat around the middle, are some of the considered reasons.

When you start, for example, with a pain in your neck, you instantly associate it with turning your head too quickly or sleeping awkwardly. You would never think about it being linked to stress or that it was your body's natural reaction, based on your thoughts to a person or situation. My next case study illustrates this problem perfectly and is about a client who came to see me in clinic with a severe pain in her neck.

CHARLOTTE'S STORY

Charlotte was a 36 year old accomplished musician. For the past 10 years she had worked as a self employed music teacher in an independent school, offering pupils private music lessons. She had a quiet personality, was very gentle, never liked aggression of any kind and was always looking for the alternative solution to a tricky situation. She came to me as she had been suffering for over three months with a severe pain in her neck, which had now started to travel down into her shoulder and affected the way she held certain instruments. She was considering some time off sick, but to prevent that, she had tried some physiotherapy as advised by her doctor, as well as some light exercise, but the problem continued to persist with the pain getting worse. It was now beginning to affect her sleep patterns as well as her mood and she didn't know how to deal with it.

After taking her medical history and completing a thorough consultation, there were no evident signs of physical trauma to her neck, shoulder or back. I could tell that Charlotte was really a healthy young woman, her pain was being created by something that was bothering her subconscious mind. As she lay face down on the treatment couch, arms to the side, I began to examine her upper back, first pressing on the right side of her neck at which point she shrieked 'ouch' at the slightest touch. Further investigations on the left side displayed tender areas, but not as painful as her right side. She had severe blockages on the right side of her neck and shoulder, which had started to limit movement as she turned her head.

As the founder of the Langellotti Tri-therapy (LT therapy as it is generally now known), I used my specialised tri-therapy method to release Charlotte's neck. At first any amount of pressure, even the lightest was unbearable, but applying the synergistic combination of my advanced muscle release technique, volcanic heat and ice marble, allowed her muscles to slowly respond, releasing the pain to a more bearable level. Visually, I could see the change and feel the muscle return to its original state. As I worked on her right side, I explained that in eastern philosophies like Buddhism, the body is energy, divided into two parts. The right side is female and the left male. The significance of this is that when treating the person as a whole (mind, body & spirit), a person has to be in constant balance on all sides of the mental, physical and emotional. Charlotte was out of balance; her right side was dominated by pain, which meant her pain was being caused by a female energy in her life. As I continued working on her deeply buried pain, the colour of her skin had changed to a dark pink and remained this colour throughout the treatment. This indicated to me that her pain was masking a conflicting issue with a negative female, which had started at least three months previous (see Fig 2).

I asked Charlotte if she had been having any upsetting issues with a female either at home or at work. At first she hesitated as if she didn't like to say, then like a moment in the confessional box, she disclosed what she had been going through. She had been bullied by one of her private senior students at school. As an only child, this pupil felt she could get away with anything. It had started with the girl making nasty remarks directly towards Charlotte when no one was around and progressed to her not practicing her pieces and then telling her mother she couldn't take the music exam because Charlotte had not been teaching her correctly. The girl's mother instantly raised a complaint to the head of the school demanding answers as to why Charlotte's teaching standards were so poor. Charlotte couldn't afford to lose a pupil as she was paid for each one that she taught, so she never challenged the girl, the mother or the head. She accepted blame for something she did not do, anything for a quite life. She was really masking the problem and by keeping it hidden, it had begun to manifest in her neck. The instrument she was teaching the pupil was the violin and the neck area is a key location to playing it. Charlotte's subconscious mind was already working to sabotage the situation; it was rescuing her in time of need. If her neck was too painful to play, she could not teach the instrument and would have to be off sick, so would have to cancel her lessons with that pupil. This was a true case of someone actually being 'a pain in the neck.'

CONCLUSION

Charlotte absorbed my findings in disbelief, yet at the same time nodding her head in agreement with everything I was telling her. She began to understand that by not facing the problem head on, she had actually created her pain. I re-booked a follow up review and advised her on homecare. One week later she came back to see me and the mobility in her neck was almost 100%. She had gone into school the day after her treatment with me and spoke to the girl in question. She made it quite clear that if she did not practice her pieces, she would not be entered for the exam and if she carried on behaving in a disrespectful manner, she would no longer teach her next term. By challenging the girl in a diplomatic way, she had taken control of the situation and finally let go of the pain. Charlotte only needed to see me that second time and her neck and shoulder pain were fully resolved. The homecare I advise my clients on, helps resolve any form of back pain quickly so that you can focus on the good things in life, not the pain.

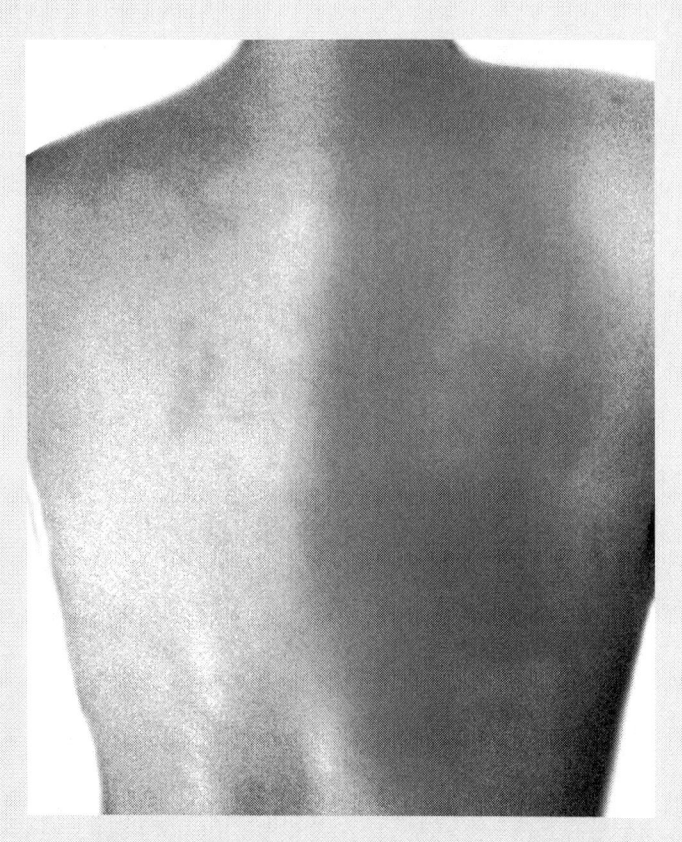

Fig 2 - Photo shows the back is darker on the right side emphasising a blockage with female energy.

3

FACT VERSUS FICTION

BACK PAIN FACTS

It is estimated that four out of every five adults (90%) will experience some type of neck, shoulder or back pain at some stage in their life. Let's look at some statistics provided by the UK government:

- In industrialised countries, up to 80% of the population will experience back pain. During any one year, up to half of the adult population (15%-49%) will have back pain.
- The number of people with back pain increases with advancing age, starting in school children and peaking in adults of 35 to 75 years of age. Back pain is just as common in adolescents as in adults.
- Back pain can range from a dull, constant ache to a sudden, sharp pain that makes it hard to move. It can start quickly if you fall or lift something too heavy, or it can get worse slowly.

- Any form of Back Pain including persistent back pain that lasts between 1 to 3 months, can have a significant impact on people's lives. It frequently reduces the sufferer's quality of life which then can affect their family and social relationships.
- Although in most cases back pain is nothing serious and disappears spontaneously, the sheer number of people affected makes it a very costly condition, imposing a considerable burden on the individual and society.
- Simple measures can be taken to reduce the chances of developing back pain and thereby reducing the impact of existing back pain.

Causes of Back Pain

- In most cases it is very difficult to identify a single cause for back pain. In about 85% of back pain sufferers no clear pathology can be identified.
- The following factors could contribute to back pain:
    - Having had back pain in the past, smoking and obesity.
    - Physical factors such as heavy physical work, frequent bending, twisting, lifting, pulling and pushing, repetitive work, static postures and vibrations.
    - Psychosocial factors such as stress, anxiety, depression, job satisfaction, mental stress.

Recovery from Back Pain

- Back pain is, in most cases, a self-limiting condition and 90% of people with acute back pain will recover within 6 weeks.
- Up to 7% of people with acute back pain will develop chronic back pain. These chronic patients have considerable discomfort and account for approximately 80% of the social and health care costs.

The Treatment of Back Pain

- Around 40% of back pain sufferers consult a GP for help; 10% visit a practitioner of complementary medicine

(osteopaths, chiropractors and acupuncturists).
- When experiencing back pain it is very important to stay active. Bed rest will only make the pain worse.
- Physical exercise can be a very effective method to reduce the pain and discomfort that long-term pain sufferer's experience. Always check with your GP if unsure before participating in physical activities.

Who Gets Back Pain?

Anyone can have back pain, but some things that increase your risk are:

- Getting older- Back pain is more common the older you get. You may first have back pain when you are 30 to 40 years old.
- Poor physical fitness- Back pain is more common in people who are not fit.
- Being overweight- A diet high in calories and fat can make you gain weight. Too much weight can stress the back and cause pain.
- Heredity- Some causes of back pain, such as ankylosing spondylitis, a form of arthritis that affects the spine, can have a genetic component.
- Other diseases- Some types of arthritis and cancer can cause back pain.
- Your job- If you have to lift, push, or pull while twisting your spine, you may get back pain. If you work at a desk all day and do not sit up straight, you may also get back pain.
- Smoking- Your body may not be able to get enough nutrients to the disks in your back if you smoke. Smoker's cough may also cause back pain. People who smoke are slow to heal, so back pain may last longer.
- Inactivity - Almost a third of young people now suffer from chronic back pain as a result of increasingly sedentary lifestyles due to computers, laptops & gaming.
- According to new consumer research, conducted on behalf of the British Chiropractic Association (BCA) 65% of 16

to 34-year-olds have experienced neck or back pain and almost a third (28%) have lived with the pain for up to a month at a time.
- The BCA warned that young people are suffering from back and neck pain as a result of leading sedentary lifestyles.
- Two fifths of sufferers said the majority of their time at work was spent "mainly sitting" and a third (32%) admitted that their back pain could be triggered by sitting still for long periods of time.
- Some 68% said back or neck pain had prevented them from exercising and sleeping and 22% had been unable to socialise with friends and family as a result of their pain.

The facts and statistics clearly show a physical link to back pain, but let's look at the bigger picture. Back pain in any form is on the increase. It's the silent epidemic of the 21st century, as stress levels grow so do our physical pains. I always say that the physical pain we feel is secondary, as the cause originates from an emotional reaction in the subconscious mind. Many people carry belief systems instilled from childhood. Belief systems are learnt from the age of 3 to 12 years of age, then we start to form our own in adolescence. But the early stages are crucial in moulding us into the adults we become. These belief systems can make or break you, and they are the foundations of the decisions you make that shape your life. They are the beliefs of your parents and what their parents taught them. Great if they work for you, but not so great if they have a negative impact.

It never fails to surprise me why we struggle to accept who we are and say 'I love you' to ourselves in the process. Love equals respect and when we respect ourselves we can love and respect others. We stand up for what we believe to be right. When I see clients suffering different levels of back pain, they all hide behind the character they have created. When they are on the therapy couch, believe me your back cannot hide the cause of the pain. I will always find it and it will always originate from an emotion, the reaction to an event or person in their past or current life.

KATH'S STORY

Kath was a woman who was always in control of everything in her life. She was a volunteer for a bereavement charity, supporting people in their hour of need. She was seen as the rock of the family. Married to Phillip for 42 years with a son & daughter, she had what some would call, a perfect life. Great health, fabulous looks and an amazing figure, especially for a woman of her mature years. As a Holistic Practitioner, I had been treating her with various complementary therapies once every four weeks for balance and relaxation. She told me during her sessions, that her husband's ongoing grumbling stomach pains had ended in an emergency appendix removal. Unfortunately, due to his age and complications from the operation, he was very poorly and recovery took six months. Kath was there, like Florence Nightingale giving him round the clock care, making fresh homemade soups by the bucket and running the house single-handed, including all the shopping and regular man chores. She put herself second to his needs and suspended any treatments she was having with me. Phillip had been to the brink of death and back, fate had granted him another innings and Kath could only count her blessings.

Shortly after Phillip came out of hospital, Kath found out her son was going through an unexpected divorce. He had not mentioned it to her before, as he knew she already had her hands full with his dad, so waited until he was out of the danger zone before breaking his news to them. Even though Kath had two wonderfully successful children, whom she loved equally, her son always had the edge in the relationship war between parent and child. Kath once again, as expected, took the news in her stride, telling me (and herself) that life was truly a rollercoaster. Other people were far worse off than her, so she could only count her blessings and soldier on, helping her son with as much

FACT VERSUS FICTION

emotional support as he needed. To her relief, her daughter had finally found a wonderful partner equally successful as her, making Kath feel a little more secure in her life.

One day I received a call from Kath quite unexpectedly, asking to be booked in for my LT Therapy, the only treatment she had never had with me. I had treated all of Kath's family on many occasions with LT therapy and they tried to encourage Kath to have a session, but she never booked. Now when everything in her life seemed to be returning to routine, with her son more settled and her husband's health almost 100% back to normal, they were even contemplating booking a holiday to their favourite place abroad to celebrate the New Year, one they had believed they would never see together. Regardless of the reason why, Kath knew it was time to have the treatment.

During her consultation, I discovered that Kath had been waking up for the last six weeks with a pain radiating from under her left shoulder which seemed to be spreading towards her spine. She thought it might be linked to her digestion, as every time she had a meal she experienced some form of indigestion and then pain followed in that area. Even though the pain had been there for a while, she left it thinking it would go away, but instead it got worse, it became sharp on the intake of breath followed by a dulling sensation. I mixed a blend of essential oils to match her emotional state of mind and compensate for her physical pain. As I started the treatment, I could feel major muscles had become blocked due to the impact of crystallized lactic acid. This forms when the person produces more adrenaline and cortisol then required, the excess converts to lactic acid and builds over time forming knots. The bigger and deeper the knot, the longer it has been there. As I explained my findings to Kath, I told her what I believed it to be, stagnant male energy that was affecting almost the whole length of the left side of her back. Again, this double whammy reflected male energy; I felt it was the nursing of her husband's illness coupled with her son's painful divorce that had shocked the family and was at the source of her pains. Clients usually listen and respond as they agree or disagree with my theory, but this time Kath was quiet. Her breathing became long and shallow and she was completely silent. I had hit the 'nail on the head' as they say; she was releasing twelve months of pain in a flood of silent tears, as if she felt ashamed of letting go. Her body was allowing her to free her pain and my stones were travelling through her muscle groups gently, but effectively deep, cutting out the toxins in order to bring back balance to mind, body and spirit. I respectfully let her get on with what she needed to do, whilst I got on with what I had to do. I followed her breath and applied my beautiful stones that worked to naturally release all the pain that Kath had stored and believe me, there was a lot of it to release. Here was a woman, a mother and a wife, who was coping with the loss of her son's marriage, the shock at almost losing a husband, her lifelong friend and soul mate. She couldn't begin to share the pain with anyone as it was her limiting belief that they would not understand. They would then have to share her pain, constantly quiz her about the state of play of things, forcing her to talk about it when that was the last thing she wanted to do - but really, deep down it was what she desperately wanted to do. Again, a classic example of how the subconscious mind controls the body to believing the opposite of what it wants. A lot like women who lack the confidence to express what they want, so say 'no' to things, when they really mean 'yes!'

I finished the treatment with my usual snapshot of the person's back (see Fig 3). I find this a great way to demonstrate to people the physical signs of their trapped male and female energy. Kath stared at the picture without a comment.

She quietly sipped her water and then the tears began to flood down her face. She sobbed her beautiful heart out, washing away the pain of all her silent suffering, now expressed in a very loud heartfelt cry.

CONCLUSION

This is a great example of exactly how to release human pain in order to restore well-being. Some people rarely or never cry, especially men, feeling that it is a sign of weakness. Besides the biological need for tears to keep the eyes moist, healthy and fight infections, tears are the foundation for humans to show empathy, compassion and grieve for loss. Tears act as an external pressure cooker, allowing us to release anxiety, stress, and upset through a physical action. Our whole body physically releases this pain and we feel better soon after. Those that cannot show this emotion or express through tears will hold on to pain until it creates dis-ease in the body, whether long term or short.

I saw Kath a week later and she looked amazingly happy, her whole body was vibrant as if a weight had been lifted from her whole being. I loved her radiant smile, it was infectious and we both had a huge hug and laughed. She was back to being Kath again, ready to save the world, as we all do.

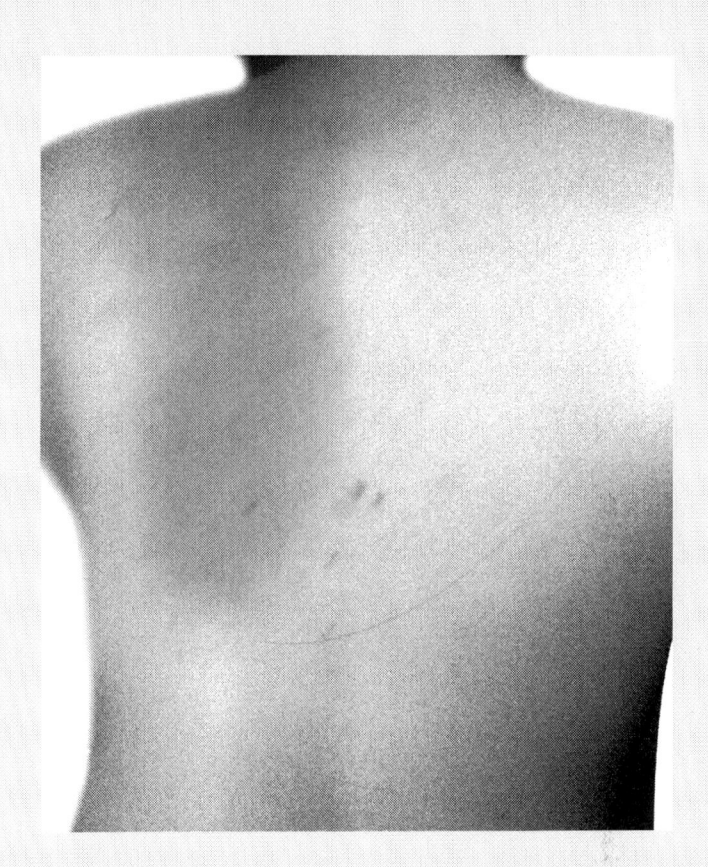

Fig 3 - Photo shows emphasis on left side male energy darker.

FACT VERSUS FICTION **41**

4

THE BRAIN

Why am I dedicating a whole chapter to the brain you may ask? Easy, our lovely brain is the control centre for our emotional & physical movement and behaviour patterns. In order to understand why we suffer back pain, we need to understand in the simplest and easiest way possible, why we do what we do to create it. So let's take a quick look at how our brain is divided and how each area functions.

The brain stimulates the head through cranial nerves, and communicates with the spinal cord that stimulates the body through the spinal nerves. The brain is like a computer, housing the location of all reason and intelligence, aspects that are responsible for cognition, mental focus, perception, concentration, memory and emotions. A developed human brain is composed of three main parts - hindbrain, midbrain, and forebrain, which are further divided into sub parts.

Brainstem

- This is the lower part of the brain where it joins the spinal cord. Almost all the nerves that come from the brain or return to the brain pass through the brainstem. The survival and arousal functions are all located in the brainstem, such as those that control breathing, digestion, being awake and alert. When the outer muscle that surrounds this area called the sternocleidomastoid muscle becomes tight, it can restrict oxygenated blood causing headaches, triggering migraines, panic attacks.

Cerebellum

- Located at the back, the cerebellum is responsible for balance and muscle coordination: movements involved in eating, walking, talking, and ability to take care of oneself.

Frontal Lobe

- As is evident from the name, it is the front part of the brain. It is one of the most crucial parts and is responsible for a person's behaviours, emotions, and cognitive abilities. The back portion of the frontal lobe is called the prefrontal cortex, and is responsible for higher cognitive functions including an individual's ability to concentrate, plan, and organize. It also determines the personality. In addition, the back portion contains the nerve cells that control and modify motor functions.

Parietal Lobe

- The parietal lobe is divided in two portions, the right area determines ability to find ways through familiar and new places, the left side is responsible for understanding the spoken and written word.
- The primary sensory cortex within the parietal lobes controls sensations of touch and pressure. A large area is connected at the back to the primary sensory cortex. Fine sensations like judgment of texture, weight, size, and shape are the responsibility of this associated area. Feeling the sensation of pain is also processed here.

Occipital Lobe
- Most of the visual capabilities are handled by the occipital lobe and the areas associated with it. It helps in visual reception and recognition of shapes and colour.

Temporal Lobe
- The temporal lobe is divided in two parts: one at either end of the brain, at about ear level. The right lobe focuses on visual memory and the left on verbal memory. Distinguishing one smell or sound from another depends upon the temporal lobe. It is also responsible for storing new information and short term memory.

You can improve your ability to perform certain functions with herbs and vitamins that promote mental fitness. However, since your brain performs dual functions, both voluntary and involuntary, it can also help in increasing concentration or mental focus. A healthy body houses a healthy mind and your brain health determines how your mind will ultimately respond to stimulations, challenges & stress.

When you suffer from back pain in any form, it is usually the secondary source not the primary cause. You have to look at the bigger picture and see what stressful challenges allowed you to manifest and eventually create the pain you now feel. Surely you may say, I couldn't make myself feel so bad, but this is how your subconscious reacts in order for you to cope with the situation.

When we are happy, in a positive frame of mind, we hold our body in a relaxed state, muscles are loose and soft. When we are angry, unhappy, feeling sad, in a negative frame of mind, we hold our body in a state of tension. The tension affects our skeletal structure, as well as ligaments and muscle groups, whether we realise it or not.

As humans, we all need love and connection, when we are challenged our brain releases the 'fight or flight' response. The fight-or-flight response is the first stage of a coordinated response called the **stress response**. The stress response involves the sympathetic nervous system, hypothalamus, pituitary gland, adrenal gland, liver and thyroid gland, which all communicate with each other by chemical messages called **hormones**.

Too much, and we have over produced copious amounts that flood our body, the excess converts to lactic acid forming knots, choosing to stay in the largest muscle groups of the body, mainly the back. When you next have a deadline to hit at work, or you are at the computer trying to finish an important document, or having a disagreement with a loved one, stop for a second to think how your body is reacting to the situation and how your muscles feel. That tension stacks up and before you know it, you are suffering neck, shoulder or some form of mid to lower back pain.

How can you prevent this you may ask? Well it's the old saying, work-life balance and everything in moderation, but in reality, it's not so simple. Twenty-first century living is moving at such a fast rate, that we can hardly keep up with the pace of life. In the 80's and 90's it was all about keeping up with the neighbours, building a family, home, great cars, fab holidays, building mega stocks and share portfolios. Then the recession hit like a Tsunami, in fact like a bus, two came along a decade apart, popping the lifestyle bubble for many. Negative equity, credit card and loan debts built to 'Everest' proportions, with people suffocating under a mountain of debt they had innocently created. Financial pressure became another 'stress factor' added to the list of life challenges.

We allow events, no matter how great or small to build inside our head, juggling between the conscious and subconscious mind. Once they reach a limit, the overspill enters the physical body, where back pain is one of the reoccurring issues we suffer. Back pain has now become known as the silent epidemic of the 21st century brought on by stress related conditions. It affects all age groups, especially younger people as more pressure is placed on the need for them to get a job as soon as they leave school/university, get on the property ladder, try to enjoy a social life including being interactive with gaming and maintaining long hours at work to prove themselves; the list goes on and affects all of us. No one can consider retirement, as they can't afford to live on any sort of pension in today's world. The only time you officially retire is when you are buried six feet under, knowing it's truly 'game over'.

MEDITATION

How common are mental health problems and do they impact the back? The following mental health facts & statistics are provided by the UK charity Mind.

1 in 4 people will experience a mental health problem in any given year. This is the most commonly quoted statistic and the one that has the most research evidence to support it.

Common Mental Health Problems;

- Depression & Anxiety – Woman have a higher prevalence of mixed anxiety and depressive disorder than men. 11.8% of the female population in England compared to 7.6% for men.
- Obsessive Compulsive Disorder – 1.3% of the population in England suffer from this disorder.
- Eating disorders – Many go unreported according to Beat (Beating Eating Disorders) suggest as many as 1.5 million people in the UK might be experiencing some form of eating disorder.
- Postnatal depression – The most common form of post natal disturbance is known as 'the baby blues' which is said to be experienced by at least half of all mothers in the western world.
- Phobias – Around 2.6% of adults in England experience phobias.
- Personality disorders- Figures range between 2% to 13% of the population in England.
- Bipolar disorder (Manic depression) – It is estimated that 20% of people who have a first episode of manic depression do not get another.

- Schizophrenia – Most studies show a lifetime prevalence for schizophrenia of just under 1%

I believe the figure to be more in the region of 1 in 3 people who will experience some sort of mental health problem in their lifetime. I see such a variety of people with varying back issues from the age of 16 to 85. Overwhelming amounts of regular stress can eventually lead to depression and anxiety, the most common mental health problems. We need to build a support system to safeguard our mind, to cope with the daily challenges. By mastering our emotional state, we ensure the physical body does not suffer and we do that by finding moments in the day, to stop and calm the mind. A few minutes of serenity in a sea of chaos has been scientifically proven to boost the brain. Too much 'chatter' in the mind is like our thoughts inside a pressure cooker. If you imagine your brain is the body's computer centre controlling every cell. Like your computer at home, it needs the junk mail emptying regularly. You organise your computer so that you can access your photos, documents and music saved in the appropriate files. When you no longer require certain data or information, you clear the file out in order to free up more memory on the computer. During meditation, there is a depth you reach in the mind where your subconscious will do this for you. Automatically deleting unnecessary negative data that no longer serves you, allowing your mind to rest and reboot itself. A healthy mind is a healthy body and vice versa. Training the mind to dip in and out of daily meditation will bring you;

- More happiness and flow in your life
- Dramatic reduction in stress and anxiety
- A greater sense of inner-peace and tranquillity
- Improved mental, emotional and physical well-being
- Heightened spirituality and a better connection with the universal energy
- Increased confidence and self-esteem
- Better, more restful and refreshing sleep
- Optimal focus, concentration and memory
- The ability to control any form of physical or emotional pain

Saying you don't have time to do it is a poor excuse. You know you do! What about all those extra minutes in the evening watching your favourite soap opera, game or talk show? They serve very little purpose, unless you want to audition to be on one! Television has its place, but can be very draining if over used. You can gain extra time in the morning by getting up 20 minutes early, allowing you to start your day in a positive way with mind-focusing meditation. You make time for your pets or your children, getting them ready for their day, don't forget the inner child in you is waiting to be recognised, valued and supported, or aren't you worth it? You may be one of those people that finds meditation difficult and prefers an alternative, like visualisation. I always say use whatever you feel works for you, but please do it! Before you give up on meditation let me say this - there are many forms of meditation, like all things in life, and you just need to find the right one that works for you. For example, I could never drink champagne, I always found it too dry or too fizzy, until one evening I attended a special event and was served the most amazing champagne. My palate exploded like the 4th July, my taste buds tingling with the most delicious flavours. I had found the right brand of champagne that had awakened my senses and released my passion for this charismatic drink.

TRANSCENDENTAL MEDITATION

Our brain, like everything we desire to master, has to be trained. Meditation is a foreign language and like all languages, we need to engage the right teacher. Attending a class speeds up the way we absorb information, so we learn meditation effectively through instruction. My quest was to find a simple, fast and effective training programme that delivered lifelong benefits and Transcendental Meditation or TM as it is known, was it. One of the most favoured forms of meditation developed 50 years ago by Maharashi Mahesh Yogi, it has been learned by over 5 million people worldwide. It is the only meditation with proven medical results. I believe when we have such powerful tools given to us by such great masters, we need to incorporate them as part of our 'work-life balance' plan. I cannot imagine my life now without it.

The David Lynch Foundation in the USA is currently bringing TM to underprivileged children in schools to help improve their education, to abused women to rebuild their confidence, to war veterans relieving post-traumatic stress disorder, to the homeless to help alleviate depression and to prisoners to address their anger, anxiety and psychological distress. In the words of David Lynch 'change starts within.' The Foundation has now extended its TM programme to the UK.

Meditation is like a colonic for the mind, when you use it daily, you are clearing out the need to store useless emotions or information that no longer serve you in a healthy way. By taking control of your thoughts and the way you tackle daily stress, you have now made room for 'work-life balance' to happen, which previously never existed. You have given permission for 'you' to be put first, in order to cope with the challenges life throws at you. Putting you first for a few minutes a day and allowing meditation to take place, means you are in a better position to help those you love the most, as you are now in control, rather than life controlling you, with endless schedules, timetables, deadlines and programmes. Even when you relax, there is always something lurking in your subconscious, so you never really switch off. By changing and training your thought pattern, you engage your powerful brain in a positive way. You welcome in the life that you truly deserve and see wonderful miracles that happen every day that you never saw before. Let's check out Melanie's story, a client of mine who lived by a limiting belief and endless agendas. By changing her thoughts and opening her mind to meditation, she experienced one such miracle.

MELANIE'S STORY

Melanie was in her late thirties and had been a client of mine for 3 years. She came to see me because of her reoccurring back pain predominantly located between her shoulders and lower back, which she associated with her job as a high flying solicitor in the city. Long hours constantly sitting at a computer, bad posture and high heels, only added to her issues. In order to ensure she stayed super slim and fit, she exercised daily following a balanced diet. She was married to Tom, equally successful, healthy and fit, who worked in the world of media. They had been trying for a baby since they got married 5 years ago, but nothing was happening. As usual, I conducted a thorough consultation, but clients do not always divulge their full emotional history to me, as they see it as irrelevant. How can the past equal the future? Well it doesn't unless things have been left untreated, then they will remain locked in the back muscles. As I said before, muscles have memory and as in eastern medicine, your back represents your past; together, they equal continuous unresolved pain.

Melanie's areas of concern were deep routed, blocking certain muscle groups around her shoulder blade and mid back. She had pressure and pain, mainly held on the right side corresponding to the female energy (see Fig 4). I often challenged her about whether she had any close female family members or friends that had caused her concern or worries for many years previous, even as far back as her childhood, but she could not put her finger on anything specific. Then one day she came for her usual monthly appointment; she had rarely practiced the homecare I had given her for the past three years, but this time she had made up her mind to rigidly follow the daily routine over the last three months. I had given her a set of specific exercises and meditations to help reduce her stress levels, stress from work that automatically had a bad habit of spilling into her personal life. I asked her to try and stop bringing her work home with her every night wherever possible, making the moments she spent with her husband more special and at the same time, healing her both mentally and physically. She was trying to create more balance in their relationship in order for her to feel relaxed every time they made love, rather than treat it as another appointment. She found it hard to shut her mind down as it counted the remaining tasks left to do, including baby-making; no wonder she wasn't conceiving!

During this particular treatment I was again looking at how her right side always seemed to build up the fastest and this had nothing to do with any physical job she was doing, it was due to an emotional blockage. On this occasion, Melanie came across more relaxed than usual, so I knew that my homecare had started to kick in, as practice makes perfect, so the saying goes. She had been meditating for a few minutes a day, shutting her chattering mind down into silence. She found it quite deep and empowering and came back more in control of her thoughts and emotions. She and Tom were enjoying their bedroom sessions more as she stopped thinking 'Is this it, the moment I conceive?'. Instead she just enjoyed the special time with Tom. Melanie would always struggle in the first ten minutes of treatment with me, as if she was hanging onto whatever she didn't want to let go of. This I feel was her subconscious mind at work sabotaging any change, but today her body had given her permission to just accept the treatment for what it was doing, releasing her muscles and allowing healing to take place. Then, when I was almost at the end of the session, Melanie said something that made my jaw drop, it was the reason for all her pain and the answer to the question I had been waiting to hear for over three years.

She started to tell me how she was beginning to really understand what I had been telling her on how controlling her stress was crucial in order to avoid her back pain building up. She started to believe, after every short simple meditation she did, that she would be blessed with a baby, she was deserving of a child and that she could finally accept that it would be easy for her to conceive. Not like in her mother's case where it had taken five difficult years to conceive her and after that, eight more years of trying for another child, that never materialised, so Melanie became their only child. Now I understood where the female blockage was, Melanie had decided that she was exactly like her mother when it came to conceiving. She believed that history was repeating itself and that her journey of having a baby was to be as difficult as her mother's, hence Melanie had not conceived in five years. I explained to Melanie that this was a break through moment, where her limiting beliefs based on her mother's experience, was sabotaging her conception. I was at no point apportioning blame, no one was at fault here, it is part of life and how as we grow, we are taught to accept a set of ideas that form our beliefs. The constant reoccurring pain on her right side was her mother's difficulties and pain in not conceiving a second child, a brother or sister for Melanie. She had listened as a child to her parent's sadness of not being able to have another baby because of their biological problems and Melanie formed her belief based on that, thinking it was part of her DNA. Melanie had now given her mind and body permission to conceive naturally, making a bold statement that she was like any another woman. It was her right to have a baby, she believed it with great conviction, she looked and felt the part, the transformation had begun.

The mind knows no limits, only those you place on it yourself. Your thoughts create fantasies, dreams, new beginnings, that are all reality to the brain, it cannot differentiate between the two. What you believe you will become, believe me it's true. Melanie had changed her limiting belief into a positive force for good. Three months later she called to tell me she was eight weeks pregnant, she had no morning sickness and no back pain; from the day she left my clinic, it never came back again and her baby was conceived. Nine months later she had a healthy 7lb 6oz baby girl and named her Sophia, after a very special lady indeed.

CONCLUSION

Melanie's story is not uncommon, it clearly outlines the power of the mind and how, when we change our thought patterns and our limiting beliefs, we change our destiny. For a few, this is easy to do, but for many they find it almost impossible to fight their demons. How much you want to change or create a new life, will determine your success to achieve it. This story highlights the fact that whatever it is you are holding onto from your past, it can be altered, as long as you recognise the need for change, forgive the hurt that was created and move on, replacing it with a positive change for good. Sometimes it's easier to live with the pain and mask the past, especially with a medical disorder that we have created and use as our crutch, to meet our need for love and connection from others. By not facing our pain or the origin of what created it, we are cheating ourselves out of a better, happier, freer life and becoming the person we were born to be.

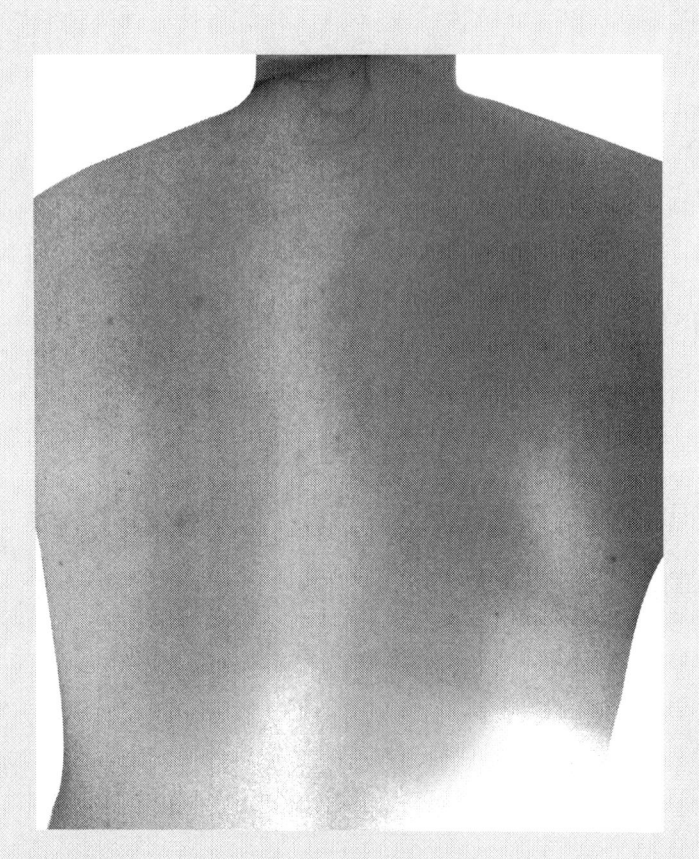

Fig 4 - Photo shows right side darker emphasising stagnant female energy.

5

FEEDING MUSCLES TO REDUCE BACK PAIN & STRESS

EAT ME DRINK ME

Alice experienced major changes when she did just what the labels asked of her, on her adventures in Wonderland. I won't be asking you to go to any such extremes in order to reduce your back pain, but I will emphasise the importance of eating and drinking right to help alleviate it. Diet not only has a very important impact on our body, but also our emotional state. There is so much information out there on how to eat right for your body, but how do you know what is right for you, especially when it comes to reducing back pain? Well, I'm not going to create the 'Back Pain Diet' that's for sure, but I am going to highlight certain things you can look out for in order to reduce inflammation in the muscles, ease aches and pains and start to feel altogether healthier all round. There are many brilliant food writers, nutritionists and chefs who support a balanced diet from maintaining perfect ph levels through to low fat, low sugar, gluten free diets, the list is endless. Through years of my own search for the 'holy grail' diet, I have found whenever I reduced stress, engaged in a healthy diet and drank more water, my back pain diminished. I asked one of the country's leading nutritionists, Fiona Kirk, who has just completed her eighth book, what makes a great diet for balancing the body's stress levels. She kindly contributed the following;

EAT TO FEED THE STRESS[1]

The word stress is regularly misunderstood. We tend to think of it as being merely an emotional thing (bereavement, money worries, work deadlines, family issues etc) but our bodies have to cope with all kinds of different stressors; emotional, physical, environmental and nutritional and the important thing to note is that the body doesn't differentiate between them - they are all seen as stress and they all trigger the same response - the adrenal glands are prompted to release the major stress hormones, adrenaline and cortisol which are life-savers when stress is short-lived but when stress is ongoing the over-activity of these hormones can seriously undermine our health.

The most common signs that the body is stressed:
- Stiff muscles and aching joints
- Poor digestion
- Erratic sleep patterns
- Allergies
- Fatigue
- Susceptibility to bugs and viruses
- Low libido or lack of interest in sex
- Cravings for sugary, salty and fatty foods

Simply put, continually-raised levels of stress hormones take their toll on the body. That 'buzz' we experience when adrenaline is racing around our system may keep us going

---
[1] 'Eat to Feed the Stress', p56-59, Source: Fiona Kirk Nutritionist

and help us to deal with the current crisis but the body doesn't like the buzz for too long and all too soon, cortisol takes centre stage in an endeavour to get a healthy balance back. We should be seriously grateful for the automatic response of this life-saving hormone but it can be the very devil in disguise when it too often arrives at the party! Elevated and untamed levels of cortisol not only prompt some or all of the above symptoms but over time can increase our susceptibility to weight gain and many of the now all-too-prevalent degenerative diseases which impede our chance of a long and healthy life; type 2 diabetes, cardiovascular disease and some cancers.

A good, balanced and nourishing diet will never be the one and only magic bullet when it comes to controlling the action of the stress hormones but it sure as hell helps.

Top eating tips

- Keep your metabolism firing on all cylinders by eating little and often and becoming a healthy grazer. Studies show that eating quality, balanced small meals/snacks every 3 hours can reduce your body's damaging cortisol levels by 20% in 2 weeks.
- Eat meals and snacks that are a good balance of carbohydrates (vegetables, whole grains, pulses and fruit), protein (lean meat, game, poultry, fish and shellfish, cheese, eggs, soya) and essential fats (oily fish, nuts, seeds) to provide the wide range of nutrients required to help your body cope with daily stressors and keep cortisol levels under control. Aim for a 50/30/20 ratio and get plenty of colour onto the plate.
- Keep the 'white stuff' to a minimum. White bread, rice and pasta, potatoes, sugar and foods/drinks with added sugars are light on fibre which means they require little digestion and are absorbed into the blood stream rather too quickly, resulting in the body looking for further

nourishment all too quickly to cope with energy dips which are yet another stress.
- Including protein in every meal and snack not only provides the body with the essential amino acids for growth and repair but also slows down the rate at which the stomach empties food into the next part of the digestive tract, keeping you feeling fuller for longer which is an added bonus if you are trying to lose weight.
- 'Good' fats are not just good, they are great. They feed the hungry brain, keep body cells flexible so they can efficiently ferry nutrients in and waste out, protect our organs, limit stress within the body, keep skin, hair and nails healthy, strengthen our bones, provide us with more energy than both carbohydrates and protein and are filling and satisfying. What's not to love! And no, great fats will not make you fat...
- If you are exercising regularly keep your glycogen (stored glucose) stores topped up by eating a balanced snack within an hour to ensure your body doesn't see the physical output as a stress and alert the cortisol devil.
- Include thermogenic foods in your daily diet. Herbs and spices turn up body heat, prompt efficient metabolism which helps to reduce stress and encourage fat burning so experiment with chilli, ginger, cinnamon, turmeric and the myriad of deeply-coloured and delicious flavours in your cooking.
- Restrict your dairy intake to natural 'live' yoghurt, cottage cheese and occasional hard goat's or ewe's cheddar and use alternative butters, milks and creams wherever possible (nut, seed, soya, oat).
- Try to sit down, relax and enjoy every meal and snack to keep those levels of cortisol under control.
- Have a treat if and when you fancy a treat to avoid dangerous feelings of deprivation but stay away from the sugary/salty/fatty varieties.
- A heavy workload, deadlines and business travel can

upset your 'little and often' eating plan big time! Try to ensure you have healthy snacks in your handbag/desk drawer/glove compartment to deal with the inevitable energy dips which the body regards as another stress and in steps the cortisol devil again. Little bags or trays of baby raw vegetables, baby tomatoes, carrot sticks, sliced or chopped fruit, small pots of hummus, tzatziki, cottage cheese or guacamole, Marigold vegetable bouillon powder and sachets of Miso soup, fruit smoothies, natural 'live' yoghurt, cold boiled eggs, chicken portions, fresh prawns, fishy sushi, mini wraps, bean, rice or lentil salads from the deli counter, mini oatcakes and rye crackers, mini cheese portions, fresh dates stuffed with almonds or pistachios, packs of raw nuts and seeds, mixed olives with feta, fruit and herb tea sachets, bottles of tomato or vegetable juice, water, water and more water!

- If you have trouble sleeping or regularly wake up in the middle of the night and can't get back to sleep it is likely that your blood sugar has taken a dive. Don't deprive yourself - good sleep is important for de-stressing the body. Foods that are rich in the amino acid, tryptophan encourage the production of the 'sleepy' chemical serotonin, so around half an hour before bed, have a couple of oatcakes with cottage cheese and/or cooked turkey, a small pot of natural yoghurt with a couple of dates, a cup of hot chocolate with soya milk and rich, dark chocolate granules or a couple of Ryvita with almond butter.

MAKING YOUR MEALS MATTER

I grew up in a house where both my parents had a passion for food, They enjoyed bringing the rich qualities of their nation's cuisine to our table, recreating colourful dishes packed with vitamins, antioxidants and minerals which enhanced our diet. I learned with enthusiasm to create those amazing flavours in my own home, so we all continued to appreciate and benefit from my heritage. Unfortunately, not everyone can say the same, food for us was an extension of our love and my mother lovingly and proudly prepared it daily for us, to share together at the table. This part of dining in today's home is sorrowfully diminishing, as families no longer are able to share meals together at the table.

Work commitments, split shifts, after school clubs, put pressure on parents to produce a fresh, balanced meal. Children get used to convenient ready made meals, eating on trays in front of the television to fill the gap of silence, watching advertisements to increase and encourage their appetites, replacing the parent and any shared conversation.

I am not for one minute apportioning blame, I can fully empathise with parents who have to juggle getting a meal on the table before running out the door to get to work. I have been there myself, but a little preparation does go a long way. I used to get ahead by using my slow cooker, a great piece of equipment, inexpensive to buy and cheap to run. From my slow cooker, the simplest but delicious dishes would materialise from the cheapest cuts of meat and vegetables, nothing in my fridge every got wasted. I used to get up thirty minutes earlier every day to prep the pot, and then set it on low, flicked the switch on, guaranteeing me a hot tasty meal when the family got home. I still use one today, when I am limited on time as there are hundreds of recipes to make, so you never get stuck producing the same thing. I encourage everyone to buy one and have fun making some great dishes, adding your own twist. You can't go wrong regardless of what you throw in, it's a one pot wonder. Adding key ingredients to your pot, as shown below, will help reduce your back pain and stress levels, as you're taking the pressure out of having to think about what to cook when you get home .You'll also feel proud that you have produced a healthy meal for all the family without it costing the earth. Most people see no relation between what they eat and their back pain. Your body needs proper nutrition so that the muscles can continue to move and support the spine. If you have not eaten regularly and sensibly, your back muscles may stop working for you; they can weaken, tighten up, and become more susceptible to fatigue-related injury and emotional stress.

EAT POWER FOODS

Your muscles need food to maintain their vigour, but not just any food. The kind of food you eat matters. In our fast-paced society, eating right can be difficult. Fast food may satisfy your hunger and may even give you an energy boost, but your muscles and your body need power foods. Power foods are the ones that provide a great deal of energy slowly, over the course of a few hours. They can keep your muscles constantly supplied with the fuel they need to maintain the support and protection of your spine. Power foods are high in complex carbohydrates and low in simple sugars and fat and contain an adequate amount of protein.

Vitamins and minerals are also important; they play a critical role in your body's ability to release the energy from foods and in keeping your body healthy. Remember to get enough calcium and vitamin D to keep your bones strong and resilient. A lack of vitamin D, the "sunshine" vitamin, may contribute to back pain. In one study, more than 80 percent of people between 15 and 52 with chronic low-back pain were deficient in this vitamin—and when they started supplementing, their back pain improved.

Try to make fresh fruits and vegetables, whole-grain cereals, whole-wheat breads, and different forms of noodles and pasta the majority of your diet. Don't drown these foods in sauces, butter, dressing, or other forms of fat. Finally, limit soft drinks, chocolate bars, ice cream, biscuits and other sweets, because they provide too much energy too quickly for the body to use. Many times, this excess energy gets converted into fat and stored in your body in places you probably don't want it.

KEEP HYDRATED

It has been proven through various studies that over 50% of the UK population are chronically dehydrated. People often mistake their thirst for hunger and choose food over water. They go about their busy lives without realising how little water they have drunk that day. A lack of water is the number one trigger of daytime fatigue and headaches. Humans are made up of approximately 65% water, this percentage varies between males, females, age and physical build.

Water lubricates our joints. The cartilage tissue found at the end of long bones and between the vertebrae of the spine hold a lot of water, which serves as a lubricant during the movement of the joint. When the joints and cartilage are well hydrated they move freely. When dehydrated the 'abrasive' damage is increased resulting in joint deterioration and increased pain. Back pain is frequently alleviated with hydration.

The need to drink more water throughout the day is a must for a zillion reasons, such as de-stressing the body, regulating temperature, increase in energy, nourishing & anti-ageing for the skin, keeping headaches away as the brain is over 75% water! I know most of you don't like it, but if you grow to love it, you won't suffer the consequences of dehydration and the suffering it brings with it.

STAY ENERGIZED

Some people eat the right kinds of food, but they don't eat frequently enough to maintain their energy level and keep their back muscles working. The most important meal of the day is breakfast, because as you sleep, the energy stored in your liver is depleted by the brain and other organs. When you wake up, about 95 percent of this reserve is gone. Your muscles and the rest of your body are just about to run out of energy and weakened muscles can quickly become injured muscles. So eat a good breakfast, and give your body and back the energy they need for the morning.

Now that you've started the day energized, you must maintain your energy levels throughout the day. The body actually works better and weight control is easier if you eat meals when you are hungry. You are probably conditioned to think that after breakfast, you should not eat until noon. However, your body may actually need the energy mid-morning so if you wait until noon, you are starving your body for two hours and increasing the risk of a fatigue-related injury. This does not necessarily mean that you should eat constantly all day, nor does it mean that every time you are hungry you should sit down to a full meal. A slice of whole-wheat bread, a piece of fruit, or some low-fat yogurt may work just fine to keep your energy up and tide you over until you can have a complete meal.

Most people still believe in the three-meal diet, but a normal body should actually consume five or six small meals per day rather than two or three large ones. Research has shown that the routine of smaller, more frequent meals is much more effective in meeting the body's energy needs and reducing the storage of body fat than the traditional three-meal diet. Just be sure that you choose healthy foods for your six small meals.

Eat more

- Cherries - One study showed that drinking 12 ounces of cherry juice twice a day for eight days reduced muscle pain and strain. Fresh or canned cherries are also helpful
- Olive oil
- Canned salmon, sardines packed in water or olive oil, mackerel, albacore tuna, flaxseed, and walnuts - all good sources of omega-3 fatty acids
- Vegetable protein (such as soy)
- Vegetables and fruits (canned or frozen are fine, as long as they're not packed in heavy syrup or loaded with salt)
- Nuts of all kinds
- Green tea
- Ginger - Try steeping a bit of grated root in boiling water with a slice of lemon for an excellent detox in the morning
- Dark leafy greens fight oxidative stress
- Avocado - high in vitamin K with pain-reducing properties
- Acai
- Turmeric

Eat less

- Certain vegetable oils such as corn, safflower, sunflower, cottonseed, or "mixed" vegetable oils
- Processed foods
- Foods high in saturated fat, including meat, tropical oils, and full-fat dairy products
- Foods made with trans fats
- Gluten
- Egg Yolks - contain arachidonic acid which can cause inflammation
- Meat, in particular red meat
- Milk, dairy
- Beer
- Fried foods

Help to minimise your back pain by cutting out or reducing foods that raise inflammation in the body and introduce more clean foods that support and de-stress the body. My next case study shows how one of my clients did just that, with incredible results.

MONICA'S STORY

An accomplished International harpist, Monica travelled the globe touring with the world's greatest orchestras. She was 32 and at the peak of her career. Graduating with honours from the Royal Academy of Music and Le Conservatoire Paris, she had been coming to me for back treatments for two years at my Harley Street Clinic. The weight of lifting her harp and driving up and down the country to perform up to ten concerts a week, was taking its toll on her slim, tall build. She seemed more like a ballerina than a musician and you could hardly imagine her transporting such a cumbersome instrument, but she did. I constantly advised her on changing her diet to reduce inflammation on the body, in particular her back, as her 'yo-yo' dieting of grabbing what she could on the run and lack of hydration was leaving her energy resources depleted. She also was unhappy that her long term boyfriend Paul, who she lived with in London, was not making the commitment she had expected by now. She wanted the proposal and her discontent was reflected on the male side of her back, in the form of pain radiating from under her scapula (see Fig 5). As fast as I could remove it she was creating it, we were like a cat chasing its tail, at logger heads to go forward. She would not settle until she had the ring on her finger. I was no fairy godmother and I couldn't produce a magic wand to make Paul propose, but I could challenge Monica to change her diet, including drinking more water for four weeks, to see if raising her energy levels would have a balancing effect on her moods and stop her from getting this build-up of pain.

When Monica returned four weeks later, it was like she had had her epiphany. Her skin was radiant and glossy, eyes alert and she literally bounced into my clinic. Something had clicked and a change was evident. She had a Cheshire cat grin and I almost believed that Paul must have proposed, but shockingly he hadn't. 'You were so right' she beamed, 'I feel sensational and have so much energy. I sleep better and I don't feel the same amount of pain as I did before'. Monica had started the 'Clean Program & Detox Diet' by Dr Alejandro Junger MD. I checked her areas of concern and there was tightness, but it was minimal compared to how it was previously. Monica then launched into her revolutionary dietary changes, which included drinking super green juices, as well as eating several small fresh healthy meals throughout the day. She had a good breakfast every morning, not like before when she used to miss it. She cut out all caffeinated drinks including the great British cuppa she loved and coffee- no more Costa. She took vitamin & herbal supplements including Omega 3-6, Chlorella super greens & a daily multivitamin. She drank boiled water with lemon juice in the morning, followed by 2 litres of filtered water a day. She hadn't had any arguments with Paul for a month, which was a first, so her moods had definitely become more balanced as she became more chilled. She learnt to cook fresh, simple basic meals, instead of eating the ready-made trays from the supermarket. She finally understood what I had been telling her for the past two years and like a jigsaw puzzle, all the pieces were beginning to fall in to place. She continued to stick to her new regime over the next six months, noticing continued improvements especially reduced pain in her back. On Christmas Eve 2012 at midnight, Paul proposed to Monica in her home city of Paris, by the Eiffel Tower. He was a true romantic at heart, but their years of squabbling made him hesitant for a full commitment. Seeing the changes in Monica gave Paul the reassurance and confidence to make that commitment.

CONCLUSION

Paul was seeing the real Monica now, whereas before he saw a stressed-out woman who lived off fast food and processed meals. This type of diet brought out a more stressed Monica and like a vicious circle, the more you feed the body with toxic foods the more the body craves for it. It brought out the moody side of Monica, upsetting the balance of hormones leading to disharmony in the 'whole' self, mind, body and spirit. By making those key changes, Monica was introduced to a side of herself that she had not seen before, and she liked it. If you truly want to reduce pain and inflammation in the body, you need to address your diet and it is very hard when you are set in your ways. As we get older and the daily demands of life stacks up against us, we just want to grab the nearest pleasurable food or drink we can imagine, whether it's sweet or savoury without thinking of the consequences. Emotional eating is one of the main reasons we struggle with obesity in the UK today, children eating processed foods due to low income families, teenagers suffering eating disorders and adults using it as a tool to fill the void in their lives and cope with emotional stress. It's not difficult to change, you just need to be committed to do it and decide why you want to in the first place. Once you make that decision extraordinary changes will occur, as in Monica's story, the magic really did come true.

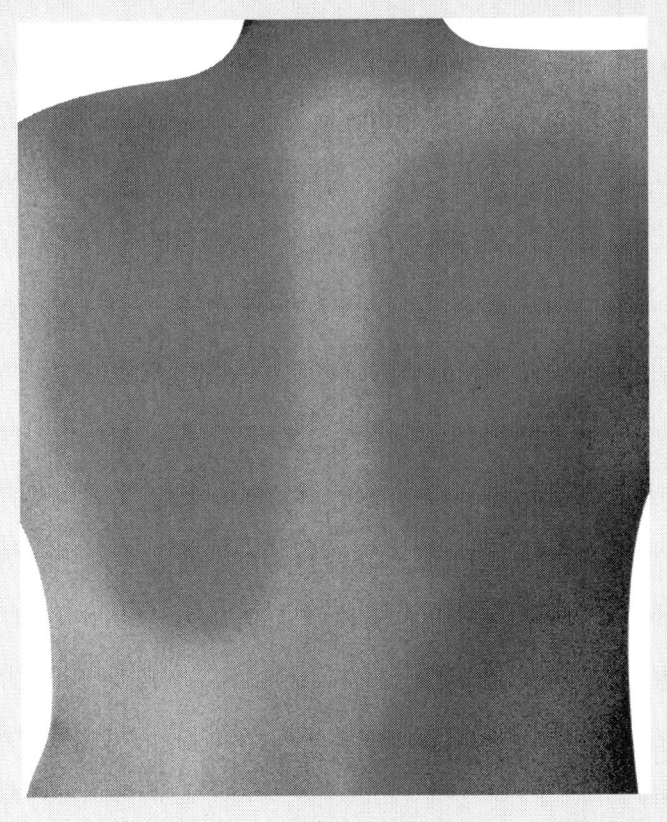

Fig 5 - Photo shows darker left side emphasising blocked male energy.

6

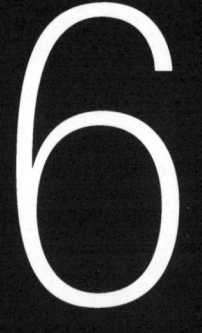

EXERCISE - DO YOU OR DON'T YOU

We know the importance of exercising, but as soon as we start with back pain, do we or don't we carry on with our activities? The simple answer is, use your common sense. If you are in incredible pain, absolutely not and check it out with your GP. If it's mild to moderate, take control with appropriate pain killers and continue with gentle exercise which benefits the brain, allowing us to de-stress. Exercise though for many, is a 'no go' area for numerous reasons; poor mobility, weight gain, illness, time poor, financial difficulties and whichever other reasons you would like to add to the list, please do. When I was at school many moons ago, physical education was compulsory on the curriculum, as it is today, however, budget cuts mean children do not get as many hours as I did to do physical activity at school and parents are left to carry the expense, using after-school clubs to extend their children's sport and dance programme. For those families on a low income, this unfortunately is an unaffordable option, so many generations miss out on the continued benefits of exercise and the importance of keeping active for a healthy mind and body. Taxiing our children everywhere, which didn't exist in the 60's 70's, or 80's means they do less walking, so their backs become less resilient. Is it any wonder our nation starts suffering at a young age from back pain, when they have to carry school bags the size of a medium suitcase filled with colossal text books. Their backs can't cope, they suffer with droopy shoulders, neck ache, headaches and referral pains elsewhere, affecting their posture in later life.

I stopped taking regular exercise myself when I left school at 18, having a natural, slim build and officially being classed as underweight, I never saw the need for it. I kept myself busy walking everywhere, doing daily housework, as well as pacing around the large office I worked in as a junior clerk. I was burning off any extra calories without realising it and at the same time, keeping my back muscles strong and toned due to a healthy diet and stress free life. That was 1980, fast forward today, in just over thirty years the pace of life is unrecognisable. Gym memberships are popular as ever, but as members we have a regular 'stop start' attendance record, depending on the season, the weather and of course what's happening on our daily agenda that breaks the routine. Most people (me included) don't like gyms, as they are boring, and why do people who don't like gyms form this opinion? We are all promised a sensational training programme, tailor-made to fit our needs when we join, but we soon realise that the friend we signed up with can't go as often as originally planned, or our individual plans change and we've already broken that New Year's resolution we promised ourselves, to get fit and keep healthy. However, friend or no friend, you still make the effort and carry on, becoming like all the others, a lonely hamster on the treadmill, bike, cross-trainer, barely speaking to anyone, just acknowledging with a glance, checking out the designer gym gear and whose physique is filling it. The only sound you can hear is the booming pump music and grunting vocals from over strained groins. Soon boredom sets in, as we don't quickly see the results we were hoping for, our motivation and goodwill is lost and we crash and burn our way out of the membership.

REBOUNDING

In September 1983 at the age of 20, I had the opportunity of visiting my godfather in Toronto Canada. It was more than a holiday, I was there to see whether I could build a career and new life in this very prosperous country. He had made the move from England, after meeting his wife and within 15 years had built a very successful business in his new home town. I was filled with excitement at the prospect of having the same amazing chance. I distinctly remember the day I arrived; it was late afternoon and Jean his wife, told me that my godfather Michael was waiting for me in the lounge, located in their basement. I eagerly ran down the stairs to greet him and couldn't believe what he was doing when I got there. He was bouncing very gently on a mini trampoline in his socks, shorts and t-shirt. 'Don't stop' I shouted, 'please finish what you are doing, then we can say a proper hello.' He shouted 'thanks' and continued for a further five minutes. When he had completed his exercise he hopped off the equipment and gave me a big sweaty hug. He had just completed 20 minutes of non-stop bouncing without lifting his feet off the trampoline and he wasn't even breathless, yet his whole body had been worked to the core. I had never seen a mini indoor trampoline before, especially one used by an adult and was intrigued as to what he was doing with it. He explained that two years previous, after a lifetime of zero exercise, he suffered a massive heart attack that almost killed him. Long hours at work to build his flourishing business made him time poor and with it came a fatty diet of fast foods at work and late night meals at home. His consultant said he was very lucky to be alive and placed him on a strict diet and exercise plan. The mini trampoline exercise programme was very well established in the USA and Canada, known as 'Rebounding.' Now the bouncing action I mistook as a grown adult being childish, had turned out to be a very serious exercise indeed. He went on to explain the vast benefits rebounding had on the whole body, keeping weight under control, strengthening the heart, boosting the immune system, supporting joints and excellent for building back muscles & core strength. Wow! Why wasn't this incredible piece of equipment available in the UK and if it was, how come I had never seen it before or heard about it? Over the next three weeks, I enjoyed the huge benefits of the mini trampoline, but found that when I returned to England, I could not get hold of one at all. Yes outdoor, but not indoor. I never had enough points to qualify and immigrate to Canada, but my journey had not been in vain. 15 years later, when my son was six years old, the mini trampoline became his life saving apparatus.

Alex my son and second child, was born with Dextrocardia Situs Inversus, meaning his internal organs were completely reversed, opposite to what we usually class as normal. In May 1993, when he was born, he was readmitted to hospital 24 hours after being discharged from birth. Consultants suspected his lungs were under developed as he struggled to breathe. An x-ray proved he was perfect, however he had a rare genetic condition undetected at the time of his 20 week scan. Within hours, I had five top respiratory consultants at my beck and call, as this was an extraordinary event and none of them had ever seen a child with this rare medical text book condition. The statistics were then, one in every 150,000 babies born had this genetic disorder and 50% with Dextrocardia also had Primary Ciliary Dyskinesia (PCD) which was later confirmed at the age of 7 through a nasal brushing test. This is where the cilia hairs that line the ears, nose and lungs don't function. Cilia clear our airways continually, but for those who have PCD, their cilia are abnormal, so in order to clear their airways, exercise and daily chest physiotherapy is crucial in order to prevent infections, which can eventually be fatal. Alex grew to hate his chest physio finding it boring, so in order to add variety to his daily routine, I remembered my trip to Canada and bought a mini trampoline which had now become widely available. I showed him the best way of using it and he started rebounding. Fortunately, it worked and it was to become his life saver. He bounced for 10 minutes at a time, 15 times a day. For over 10 years he was the healthiest child with PCD attending his monthly paediatric hospital clinic and the only child, to have one course of antibiotics a year, which was unheard of if you had PCD. I told the consultant what he was doing, but they sceptically rejected the idea. Alex's enthusiasm for rebounding ensured he bounced his way through one trampoline a month, which was costing me a small fortune. After much research, I imported from Germany a Bellicon trampoline and never looked back. It is now available in the UK (see back of book for more details). Alex is now a very healthy 20 year old young man and continues to rebound daily. I even bought a second trampoline which he took to campus whilst studying for his degree. Rebounding boosts his immune system, strengthens and clears his airways, supports his back, it is a total body workout.

In life we sometimes meet people or travel to places for reasons unknown to us at the time. My brief trip to Canada was never about me going to live there, it was to discover the many benefits of the mini trampoline and what rebounding had to offer, not just in my son's case. I now highly recommend it to all my clients, especially those who have medical problems restricting their movement (once they have checked with their GP), those with weight issues or those who dislike any form of exercise as a way of supporting and strengthening their back, with no impact to the knees or rest of the body. Exercise should be fun. We all need to release our inner child and rebounding certainly does that and much more.

PERSONAL TRAINING

Even though I do rebound daily, whilst researching this book I had to find out if taking part in a higher form of exercise would benefit our muscles even more and help reduce or even erase back pain. I knew from past experience that going it alone, with my own gym programme would never work, I wasn't disciplined enough to push myself. Rebounding was easy, a few minutes twice a day, was effortless and fun, but the gym was not. I decided that I needed to enlist the services of a personal trainer to work one to one with me and show me another way of keeping fit and strengthening my back. Would interval training hold the key to changing my negative approach about the gym, or would it turn out to be too aggressive for back pain sufferers? I chose a local independent boutique gym that specialised in offering bespoke training programmes to deliver real results. Sounded like it had my name written all over it, so I signed up for three months. I went through the usual weigh in, body fat percentage and inch measurement. I was introduced to James, my athletic personal trainer. He would now be my new shadow, whether I liked it or not. I had to stick to the three month contract with a six day commitment each week, in order to complete my study. I went through specific things with him that I wanted to achieve, a key one being to strengthen my legs and upper body.

I was working in London and commuting weekly from Leeds on the train. Two and a half hours sitting on the Southbound train, then facing the challenges of the Underground, finishing off with a ten minute walk to my Harley Street Clinic from Oxford Circus. Reads like a three course meal, hardly challenging you may think, but think again. When you are carrying ten volcanic and ten marble stones in your backpack, plus other tools of the trade required for my work, believe me, it's no picnic. It becomes like an army assault course with 10kg strapped on your back. I realised after six months, my lower back was beginning to tire and in order to keep up with two busy clinics, I had to make myself become super strong. I explained to James that I was five months away from turning fifty, hoping I would win the sympathy vote and he'd go easy on me, but he didn't even flinch, saying age had nothing to do with it. He would be challenging my core and boy did he do that! Rebounding was gentle, kept me toned and supported my muscles, but interval training gave me a more tailor made result at a higher level.

Three months later I went into the side room to be re-measured and tested. I had reduced my body fat by 7%, went from 63 kilos to 59 kilos (impressing my GP) without a dietary change, hit the perfect BMI and had the blood pressure of a 30 year old, reducing most of my body by a few inches everywhere. I had never looked so good and even James admitted that for a woman of my age (yes, I'm getting used to those comments now I am fifty) I was the envy of many women half my age. Even though those observations made me feel like I had just conquered Everest, my best result was my fitness level and core strength. They had increased by 100% and I had never felt so physically fit in all my life. It was like a new athletic me that I had unleashed and I was giddy about it. My back muscles were re-contoured and my legs were strong enough to run a marathon or near enough. I never believed it was possible, as I was the one who had been told that I may have to spend the rest of my life in a wheel chair, yet here I was, proving those medics wrong. I felt like Rocky Balboa at the end of his dramatic fight scene, victorious. Anything is possible and age is just a number that people use as an excuse to talk themselves out of doing things or committing to a challenge. 'Feel the fear and do it anyway' said the wonderful Susan Jeffers and by God she was right. I am always regarded as Miss Positive, but when it came to fitness and the gym, it was my Achilles heel. My real fear was being told 27 years ago after the accident, that I had a damaged sciatic nerve and I was frightened that if I pushed myself at the gym, I would open up old wounds and possibly damage it even more. This is a fear most people with back issues or injuries live with, I was one of them. If that had happened, then it was game over for me and my career. See how my own limiting belief cost me years of a high standard of fitness, allowing me to create a false reality? So I used boredom as my excuse not to go to the gym, masking the real reason, hiding my fear from everyone.

As I sat down with pride and reviewed my results, I wanted to pinpoint what had created the change in me. Easy, I learnt from the first day on my training programme that it was my mindset, coupled with a chemical change. Yes, I had felt for the very first time my superheroes kick in like never before, because I had never challenged myself to such a level. I had never experienced what I did at the end of my first session. I remember arriving on my first day at the gym, having a rush of adrenaline well before I had started to warm up. I placed my emergency remedies (to cover any possible panic or anxiety attacks) in the locker; a banana, my herbal tincture and endless tissues. Crazy thoughts began rushing through my head, like my brain was already having its own mini workout! I visualised myself leaving the gym, hands shaking at the point of passing out, unable to drive myself home because of the intense workout, my body being a wreck, even James having to do CPR on me, what a thought! Once again, see how my imagination was sabotaging my mind, 'Another reason to cancel the session' I told myself, but I didn't. What really happened after my first session was a state of ecstasy, through which my body had reached a 'natural high.' My 'feel good' hormones known as Serotonin, Dopamine, Oxytocin and Endorphin, had arrived like the cavalry, they were my 'Four Musketeers.' You get the same super hero release whilst rebounding, but at a different level.

Serotonin:
- Serotonin is the happiness hormone. Serotonin regulates our moods and keeps mood-swings at bay. It also prevents depression and anxiety. It increases happiness and a sense of well-being. Serotonin can be released by getting exposed to sunlight, by eating foods rich in carbohydrates and by exercising.

Endorphins:
- Endorphins also make you feel good and more relaxed; it also reduces anxiety and all forms of pain. Endorphins are released by moderate to vigorous exercising.

Dopamine:
- Dopamine helps with mental alertness and clarity. The lack of it causes foggy thinking and a lack of focus and concentration in addition to setting increased depression and despair. It can be released by eating foods that are rich in protein which is high in any fitness enthusiast's diet.

Oxytocin:

- Interestingly, Oxytocin is the new kid on the block and a recent discovery suggests that different types of exercise such as walking, mountain biking and aerobics can help release oxytocin into the bloodstream, reducing stress and anxiety symptoms.

How could I ever live without these guys! They were responsible for helping me maintain my happy state, balanced moods and keeping my stress in check. Without them daily, when we experience challenging events, we lose control leading to stress. This in turn makes us negative, angry and tense, allowing adrenaline to flood our body, with any excess being stored in the muscles, converting to lactic acid that eventually form knots leading to pain. The only thing to remember is that these guys show up at the point of high activity, so any activity not just exercise will do, like fast walking, brisk housework, intense gardening (I'll leave the rest to your imagination). We should try to keep up to this level of movement regularly, daily sessions would be ideal. Thirty minutes broken down into three ten minute sessions or two fifteen minute mini activities will trigger these heroes into action, so the earlier you start to be active in the day, the more you will gain from their contribution. That's why rebounding has now become so popular, as you can keep the trampoline stored indoors at home and use it daily when it suits you. Events such as National Marathons, the Tour De France and Olympic Games keep the nation focused on being active. I continue to train regularly with my Personal Trainer (PT) and have made it more affordable, by joining up with a small group of people at the gym. There are usually four to six of us that meet up and we share the cost of the personal training session, which many gyms are now starting to offer. This way, we all get a great workout and the trainer can give us enough attention individually to correct any mistakes. Successful training is more achievable for most people when they have a buddy running beside them, motivating them or a PT. If you can do it on your own and attain the same results, well done! I couldn't, but by using a PT I achieved results beyond my expectations and am motivated to continue in the long term. An experienced PT corrects you when you're doing the exercise wrong, reducing any chance of injury. A PT will always demand more of you, as they are qualified to know how far they can push your body. They will increase your weights and workload as they see you progress and when you say you can't, they shout 'YOU CAN!'

HARRY'S STORY

Harry was Head of Training at a prestigious airline operating from Heathrow Airport. He came to see me at my Harley Street Clinic in London, as recommended by his dear friend Joseph, whom I had recently treated. Harry was 48 and in fabulous shape, he was a health & fitness fanatic, taking care of his body like a temple and looked easily twenty years younger. I didn't need to lecture him on diet and exercise, he practised it daily like a religious devotee. During his consultation his only concern was the pain he had been feeling from the top of his right shoulder down through his trapezium muscle. He blamed it all on pressure at work, irregular sleep patterns because of his flight schedule and workmen outside his house, on a long term project, drilling during the day when he was trying to sleep. He had suffered this constant pain, like a dripping tap for four years and had spent £25,000 travelling the world in search of a cure. Finally, he came to me to see if my methods would instigate a change and resolve his predicament. I was amazed how early he was for the appointment, by almost 15 minutes. He then disclosed that he had been next door for an hour of Myofascial release treatment on his back. I asked him why he had chosen to have another back treatment before having my treatment, especially an hour before. He said that he didn't see the point of cancelling the other appointment and didn't think it would matter. There are three levels of 'LT Therapy' and

Harry was booked in for the middle level, which lasts one hour and incorporates some Myofascial therapy. Would he see the benefits of my treatment after already having some release work done, and would I find anything left to work on?

My back treatment starts with the selection of essential oils (in consultation with the client) which work to support their mind, body and spirit. I then commence a short ritual of touch, placing the palm of my hand down on the back, applying a light to medium pressure in order to locate the key areas that are locked. I am like a trouble shooter, assigned to annihilate toxic build-up that creates pain in acute areas, as well as extended regions of the body, which may affect the head, arms and legs. My palm undulates like a heat seeking missile, searching for its target. Like the voyages of Captain Kirk on the Starship Enterprise, my mission is to explore strange new blockages, to seek out new life in these back muscles, to boldly go where no man has gone before with 'LT Therapy.' Harry had good flexible muscles for the majority of his neck, shoulders and back which was to be expected, as he had just had some release work carried out. However, where his area of concern was, the build up was untouched; it remained an undisturbed, solid lump of tissue, as hard as concrete to the touch. As I pressed on it, his body reacted with a jump, like he had been given an electric shock, quickly followed by a painful burst of 'awah!'. Yes, his nemesis was still there. Tuning into his energy field, I could feel this was quite deep, as I started to break down the knot using a sequence of heat, ice and my advanced muscle release technique. I told him that the problem lay on his right side which represents female energy (see Fig 6). I asked him if he had lost someone very important to him around four years ago, someone like a mother figure. He replied yes, his mother whom he was extremely close to had died of cancer four years previous and his pain began shortly after the funeral.

Harry was holding onto his mother's memory, finding love and connection in his back pain. He had not dealt with her loss and was still suffering bereavement. Time is a great healer, but only if you acknowledge the death and move on. Harry was silently shielding his loss, not accepting her death. I explained to him what was happening and how his state of mind was allowing his body to carry the pain in a physical form. He totally connected with what I was saying and agreed that he had found it extremely difficult to bear on his own. His twin brother lived on the other side of the world and he had a poor relationship with his sisters. As he talked throughout the treatment, telling me about his wonderful mother and what they had shared together, he was releasing his pain. I could feel a huge discharge of negative energy like a tsunami leave his body and flexibility was returning to the muscle at lightning speed. He shed no tears as he sat up after the treatment and talked, it was like a huge weight had been lifted from his shoulders. His eyes a little glazed, he left the clinic with a follow up appointment two weeks later.

I watched Harry walk down the corridor as I went to greet him on his return appointment. The way he moved was unrecognisable, he had so much zing in his step and a great carefree swagger I had not seen before, he could easily grace a male catwalk any day. This new found lightness in his body gave me a sense of hope that something good had happened that day and there was more to come. The smile on his face was like no other I had seen before, it was as if he had seen his mother. I expressed my joy at his glowing persona and asked if he had experienced any other changes. He began to reel off like a machine gun every minute benefit the treatment had given him. From the moment he walked out, he felt his pressure lifted. He slept like a newborn baby that night which continued over the following weeks. He started back at the gym full time, where previously he had only been going two days a week and toward the end, had stopped attending altogether for fear of making his pain worse. He blamed exercise for aggravating his pain and other demands in his life, but they were only masking the truth. He was now back to being himself, living life to the full, feeling as good as 'Superman.'

CONCLUSION

Harry continues to see me once a month having 'LT Therapy' treatment as part of his 'work-life, balance' programme. Most people would blame their physical fitness regime as the cause of the pain, but for Harry the real reason was buried deep in his back and was clearly linked to the loss of his mother. It never ceases to surprise me when people walk through the door of my clinic, what I will uncover. I always say that if I was a man, I would probably have been a priest as I've always been good at not disclosing personal information or surrendering secrets. I was the Marjorie Proops at my school, as people shared their problems with me to which I offered support, keeping their confessions to myself. My client's stories are private and a reflection of their own journey. I always feel privileged when during the treatment they choose to share their pain with me. As they openly speak, they are releasing the cause feeling instantly free and experiencing a quicker recovery. As the saying goes, a problem shared is a problem halved.

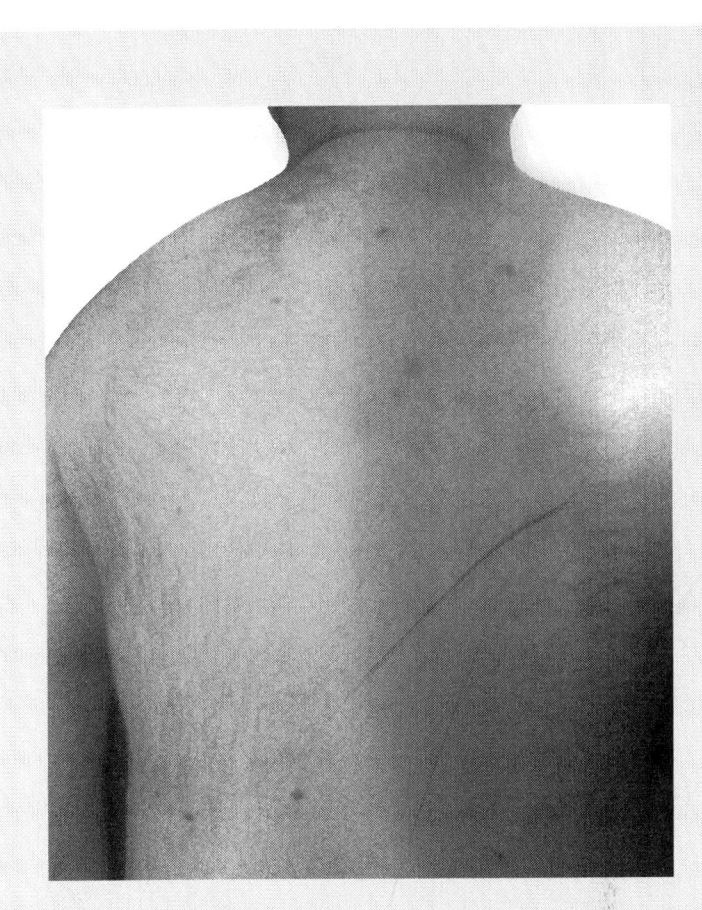

Fig 6 - Photo shows darker right side emphasising female energy blocked.

7
TAKE CONTROL

Managing pain is extremely important while the body heals and recovers. So many of us don't know what to take, when to take it and for how long for fear you may turn into a painkiller addict! One thing I did learn in the two years I worked with the pain management clinic whilst nursing my father through his final years with heart disease, was the importance of controlling pain and how it improves the quality of your life. In my 20's, especially at the time of my accident, I was against taking any form of painkillers, due to my lack of knowledge and understanding the importance of their role. In some ways, I am glad of that time of ignorance, as I discovered the power of using the mind in assisting pain control.

How does your brain know when you feel pain? How does it know the difference between the soft touch of a feather and a needle prick? And, how does that information get to your body in time to respond? How does acute pain become chronic pain? There are no simple answers, but with a little explanation about how the nervous system works, you will be able to understand the basics.

THE NERVOUS SYSTEM

Your nervous system is made up of two main parts: the brain and the spinal cord, which combine to form the central nervous system; and the sensory and motor nerves, which form the peripheral nervous system. The names make it easy to picture: the brain and spinal cord are the hub, while the sensory and motor nerves stretch out to provide access to all areas of the body similar to a motorway connecting access to towns, cities and villages.

Simply, sensory nerves send impulses about what is happening in our environment to the brain via the spinal cord. The brain sends information back to the motor nerves, which help us perform actions. It's like having a very complicated 'In' and 'Out' box for everything.

PAIN BEGINS WITH NERVES

Let's say you step on a rock. How does a sensory nerve in the peripheral nervous system know this is any different than something like a soft toy? Different sensory nerve fibers respond to different things, and produce different chemical responses which determine how sensations are interpreted. Some nerves send signals associated with light touch, while others respond to deep pressure.

Special pain receptors called nociceptors activate whenever there has been an injury, or even a potential injury, such as breaking the skin or causing a large indentation. Even if the rock does not break your skin, the tissues in your foot become compressed enough to cause the nociceptors to fire off a response. Now, an impulse is heading through the nerve into the spinal cord, and eventually all the way to your brain. This happens within a nano second.

YOUR SPINAL CORD: THE MIDDLE MAN

Your spinal cord is a complex array of bundles of nerves, transmitting all kinds of signals to and from the brain at any given time. It is a lot like a huge network for sensory and motor impulses. But your spinal cord does more than act as a message centre: it can make some basic decisions on its own. These 'decisions' are called reflexes.

An area of the spinal cord called the 'dorsal horn' acts as an information hub, simultaneously directing impulses to the brain and back down the spinal cord to the area of injury. The brain does not have to tell your foot to move away from the rock, because the dorsal horn has already sent that message. If your brain is the body's CEO, then the spinal cord is middle management.

HOW YOUR BRAIN SEES PAIN

Even though the spinal reflex takes place at the dorsal horn, the pain signal continues to the brain. This is because pain involves more than a simple stimulus and response. Simply taking your foot off the rock does not solve all of your problems. No matter how mild the damage, the tissues in your foot still need to be healed. In addition, your brain needs to make sense of what has happened. Pain gets catalogued in your brain's library, and emotions become associated with stepping on that rock.

When the pain signal reaches the brain it goes to the thalamus, which directs it to a few different areas for interpretations. A few areas in the cortex figure out where the pain came from and compare it to other kinds of pain with which it is familiar. Was it sharp? Did it hurt more than stepping on a pin? Have you ever stepped on a rock before, and if so was it better or worse?

Signals are also sent from the thalamus to the limbic system, which is the emotional centre of the brain. Ever wonder why some pain makes you cry? The limbic system decides. Feelings are associated with every sensation you encounter, and each feeling generates a response. Your heart rate may increase, and you may break out into a sweat.

WHERE IT GETS COMPLICATED

While it may seem simple, the process of detecting pain is complicated by the fact that it is not a one-way system. It isn't even a two-way system. Pain is more than just cause and effect: it is affected by everything else that is going on in the nervous system. Your mood, your past experiences and your expectations can all change the way pain is interpreted at any given time. How is that for confusing!

If you step on that rock after you have a fight with your partner, your response may be very different than it would if you had just won the lottery. Your feelings about the experience may be tainted if the last time you stepped on a rock, your foot became infected. If you stepped on a rock once before and nothing terrible happened to you, you may recover more quickly. You can see how different emotions and histories can determine your response to pain. In fact, there is a strong link between depression and chronic pain. So when we experience pain anywhere in the neck, shoulder and back, this is a secondary reaction responding to an emotional stress response created earlier.

WHEN ACUTE PAIN BECOMES CHRONIC

In this scenario, after your foot healed, the pain sensations would stop. This is because the nociceptors no longer detect any tissue damage or potential injury. This is called acute pain. Acute pain does not persist after the initial injury has healed.

Sometimes, however, pain receptors continue to fire. This can be caused by a disease or condition that continuously causes damage like pressure building up in the muscle. With arthritis, for example, the joint is in a constant state of disrepair, causing pain signals to travel to the brain with little down time. Sometimes, even in the absence of tissue damage, nociceptors continue to fire. There may no longer be a physical cause of pain, but the pain response is the same. This makes chronic pain difficult to pin down and even more difficult to treat as in the case of Fibromyalgia sufferers.

CONTROLLING PAIN

As a holistic therapist I don't like taking tablets even when I've got a headache. I will sleep it off or see it as a sign of dehydration, so will increase my water consumption. Our bodies are machines working 24/7 to accommodate our life, all it asks is that we replenish it with good nutritious food, that strengthens our organs to create energy, drink plenty of distilled fresh water to hydrate our cells and get enough sleep, so that it can repair any damage. We are an amazing work of art in motion, yet our belief systems from childhood, our peers, our education, our jobs, our relationships make us treat our mind, body and spirit so erratically with the wrong food, too much alcohol and caffeine, poor sleep patterns, etc. so there's always something out of balance inside of us. When we are good, we are very, very good and when we are bad we are just awful. Breaking up with our partners, having a heated argument, getting worked up with the neighbours, chastising the children creates deep pain in our souls that knocks you off balance. We don't like confrontation, we don't like disagreements and challenges, whilst they are there to help us grow, they are such a pain. As we associate these emotions as painful, so they begin to resonate within us and create a negative feeling. These feelings build one on top of the other, until a Vesuvic explosion occurs in the form of pain, whether dull or sharp, you feel it somewhere in the body.

I am not for one minute condoning or encouraging you to go out and stock up on varieties of pain killers, I will say this. When you start to feel deep, heavy pain in the back causing you to have limited movement, take appropriate analgesics to help the body recover. Painkillers buy your body time to recover by temporarily allowing the superficial nerves to go to sleep. When you don't feel the pain, you walk normal, sleep normal, move normal thus not creating additional problems in other parts of the body. I have seen many people walk into my clinic thinking the more dramatic they appear the better the result they will get. All they get from me is a lecture on taking control of their pain using the correct tablets. Many people don't even know what to take, so I urge them to go to their GP or Nurse Practitioner and have a chat about any back pain they are experiencing. The doctor will dispense the appropriate level of pain killers. They will ask you to review the situation and come back if the prescription is not effective enough, until they find the right one that suits you.

HELEN'S STORY

Helen was a teacher on maternity leave with her first child Katie. She was married to David who was a partner in his father's building firm. They had had a whirlwind year fitting in a new house, their wedding and their baby's birth. Before this major year of events, I saw Helen every six months to release any build up which formed mainly on her left shoulder. Her relationship with David had been a rocky one in the past, but they seemed to have resolved their differences when Katie was born. It was early Wednesday morning, an hour before my clinic started when I received an urgent text from Helen, asking me to fit her in as soon as possible. Her left shoulder had flared up and she was struggling to pick up Katie as the pain was so unbearable. As soon as she got on the couch, I could not only feel the large swelling, but visually I could see a raised area near her shoulder blade. Tender to touch, I quickly packed it with ice marble and slowly started manipulating the area. I never work on bone or inflammation, I was aiming to release any pressure that had accumulated, in order to discharge the negative energy and lactic acid build up, and ease the pain rapidly. I told Helen that I had never seen her left shoulder so bad. The left side linked to a male energy (see Fig 7) causing her grief, could she relate to it? I knew she wasn't at work so it couldn't be with a male colleague, her baby was a girl so her teething wasn't bothering her and her father had passed away a decade ago which she had come to terms with, so I deduced it had to be with her husband, but it would be up to her to disclose that to me.

Silence speaks volumes. I chose not to speak again and let Helen gather her thoughts. Suddenly, without warning, she released her anger with such force that my couch shook and she almost rolled off the bed. I continued to work around and on the area, as the muscle became pliable. I needed to get it to a putty consistency in order for her to feel it lifting. She began shouting at the way David's gambling was beginning to risk their livelihood. He had been hiding his addiction from her for several months, taking money from the family business. He decided to tell her as his father had found the discrepancy and would have brought it to her attention. This was the issue that had caused problems in their relationship a few years ago, but she thought they had resolved it. Now it was raising its ugly head again. David did suffer bouts of depression, and he used the gambling as a way of dealing with it.

I was happy to see that Helen had shared her problem with me, but she now had to learn to control it. She had barely taken any painkillers as she was still breastfeeding, hence the intensity of the pain. When I had finished the treatment, I applied a natural topical anti-inflammatory cream which would help settle the symptoms over the next eight hours. I advised her to see the pharmacist who would be able to sell her the right painkiller she would be able to take whilst breastfeeding. If by Monday she was still experiencing the same, she should see her GP. I also told her that she had to deal with her anger by speaking to David telling him that this situation could not carry on and was unacceptable. I encouraged her to get help and support for David via their doctor. It was unfortunate that she never mastered any form of meditation as it would have helped her work through the challenging situation as well as the deceit. Helen knew what she had to do, she thanked me for fitting her in, her shoulder felt much better and she had mobility back. I knew the problem would return if things were not altered.

Friday of that same week, two days after treating Helen, she sent me another text asking again to be seen that day. Luckily for her I had received a cancellation and the minimum gap between seeing a client from one treatment to the next is 48 hours. She came stating that her pain had subsided after I had seen her, she did get appropriate pain killers from the pharmacist, but when she woke up this morning her pain was back again. I explained that she hadn't really given her pain killers a real chance to kick in, she hadn't taken control of the situation with David and was just suffering a panic attack. When I re-checked her back, the area I had treated had not come back. The pain had actually moved to a different area, still on the left hand side. It was amazing how the power of the mind had moved the problem elsewhere. I asked her if she had had a chance to speak to David, she said she hadn't, she was too scared of the consequences just in case he got violent. He became very withdrawn, moody and angry, raising his voice and shouting when anyone challenged him on the topic. I can tell how intense someone is feeling by the way the blockage builds and Helen was on a real low. I did release it again, this time I strongly advised her to see the doctor first thing Monday morning. I could only go so far with my treatment, for as fast as I took it away she would re-build it. She needed prescription anti-inflammatories and a referral for David, if only he would go with her.

Three months passed before Helen contacted me again. David had gone with her that Monday to seek help and was having counselling. The gambling had stopped burning a hole in their finances and she felt she could take control of the 'free falling' situation. She didn't know how long the cork would stay in the bottle, but she was going to make sure that David would not be releasing his gambling genie if she could help it. They both went on to attend a Transcendental Meditation (TM) seminar and booked to do the training course.

CONCLUSION

Helen was determined to take control of her pain and David's gambling. He was creating an insecure world for her and their daughter which she could no longer tolerate. Her back pain spiralled out of control as she went into free fall. Seeing me allowed her to put the brakes on the situation, helping to diminish her pain, giving her time to think clearly, sensibly and in a controlled manner. When someone rocks your world to the core and you lose control, the impact affects everyone around you; your children, parents, brothers, sisters, friends. By hiding your pain emotionally and 'putting on a front' the pain will manifest in the physical. If not in your back, it will find another vulnerable place in your body until you acknowledge the problem and work to resolving it. Life is like a board game with many hidden challenges, happiness and sadness is all on the shake of a dice. Learn to take control by placing exercise, diet and TM at the heart of your 'work-life balance' programme, then even when you are thrown a major disaster, you'll have the capability to handle it with surprising strength.

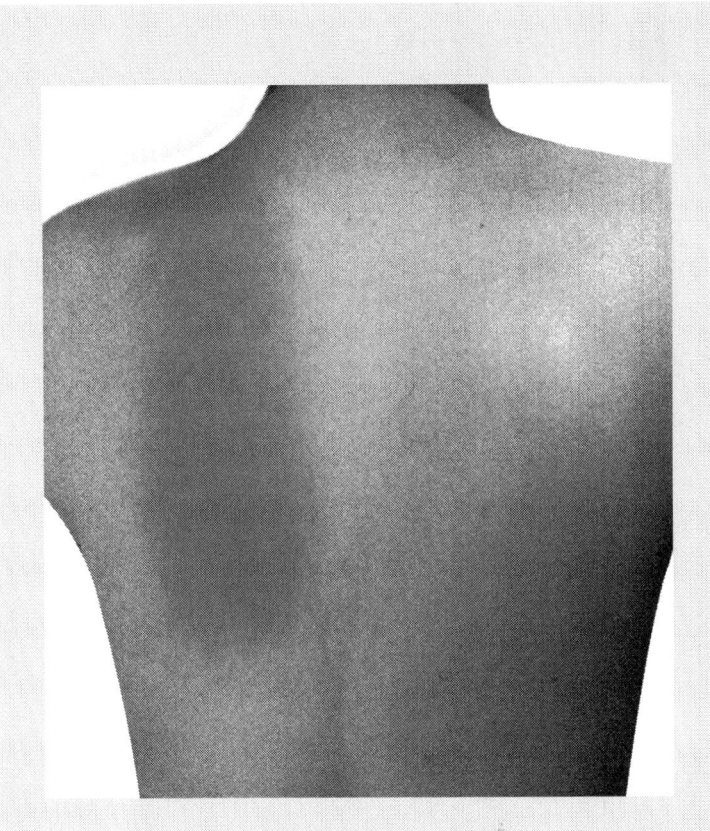

Fig 7 - Photo shows darker left side male energy blocked.

8

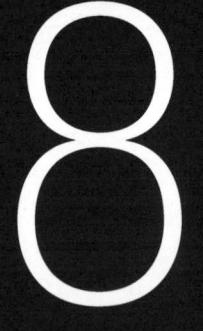

THE KEYS TO UNLOCKING YOUR BACK PAIN

In life there are many recipes for a successful outcome. Whether you are baking a cake, constructing a claymation, building a business, planning a wedding, assembling a 1000 piece jigsaw puzzle, it always starts with a plan that has to be executed in order to achieve a winning result. First, decide what has to be targeted, then pull together the key ingredients required to fit the task. In unlocking your back pain, the key to resolving it is you. You control your life and how you react to daily situations. There are certain circumstances we come across that we can plan for, like funerals, weddings, birth of a baby etc. so we are prepared. There are many things that happen which we cannot prepare for, like going to work and being challenged by a colleague or your boss, going to the doctors for a routine check up and unexpectedly being referred for further tests. A loved one suddenly being taken ill, your car breaking down, the bus not showing up, the flight being delayed; the list is endless. You've heard of the saying 'Fail to prepare, prepare to fail' so you have to prepare yourself to face the modern world. You have to install a system that is tailor made to suit your needs and will support your 'whole' self, that's the emotional, physical and spiritual side, whether you care to acknowledge it or not. Through my work, I have discovered a system which when applied, will definitely give you the means to control your 'whole being' to live a wonderful pain free life.

WHAT LIFE MEANS TO YOU

Like a 'Pick and Mix' counter, I have listed the ideal recipe for you to unlock your back pain and create a great life for yourself and loved ones. You can sample everything on offer and then incorporate all elements into your life or just add the ones that work for you. Remember, there is no wrong answer, whatever decision you make is always the right one. Whatever point you are at in your life, it should always flow. Like musical notes, we write our own life score. You can make it sound as dramatic as you like or as soft and gentle as a lullaby. I have spent the past fifty years of my life, learning and practicing how to play the game of life. I have in no way mastered it, but I'm going to spend the next fifty making sure that I enjoy putting all my life lessons into practice. Take pleasure in each day, whatever it brings you. Sometimes we sit back observing, waiting to join the merry-go-round and other times we go head first, like a bull in a china shop. Life should be embraced, fill it with passion and excitement, but then give yourself time to reflect and recharge your batteries. Let's put things into perspective. Never forget, life is beautiful, even when we suffer, someone else's pain is greater. Take no one and nothing for granted and always be grateful for the day, there is no guarantee you will get another.

I love food and I am always creating new recipes. I like playing with ingredients and experimenting with flavours, that's what you should be doing with life. Taking a blank canvas and building the most beautiful picture that reflects the best of you. What you put into life is what you get out and it will show in your painting. Do you want a Dorian Gray or Di Vinci in your attic? Another pressure society puts on us unnecessarily, is judgment. People are always judging you, even before they meet you. This falls under the category of envy, one of the seven deadly sins.

As a Virgoan, mother earth type, I was always told that I came across too serious, had high standards and chased perfection. See how people can read you wrong! I do like nice things, a comfortable home, good manners and standards. Why not, they don't cost anything and go a long way in telling someone about you. However, I am playful, fun, have a wicked sense of humour, I'm honest, loyal, reliable, and dependable and a safe bet. You can always count on me to be there for support. Trust and respect are key to me. I used to be bothered about what people thought of me but age has a wonderful way of taking those concerns away. I know the people who really know and love me, get the real me. I stopped worrying instantly and noticed that I didn't carry any pain in my shoulders like before. Not because I stopped caring, because I stopped listening to people whose opinions no longer mattered to me, and that was a weight off my shoulders.

MINI LIFE LESSONS

Don't allow anyone's negative opinion to affect you. There are no limits in life, only the one's you place on yourself. Don't blame someone else for your shortfall. Accept responsibility and move on. I brought my children up on these values and I am proud of how wonderful they have turned out. We beat ourselves up if we are not the perfect parent, but who is? Relationships, now that's a difficult one, staying with a long term partner for the sake of family, finance or work commitments. You have to be honest with yourself and put yourself first. Wow! That's a change coming from someone with a Roman Catholic background who believed that 'marriage is for life.' Well it still is, but when we make a commitment to our partner, what happens when one grows and the other doesn't? What do you do when one person loves and embraces life and the other just gives up on it? Do you owe them the rest of your life because of a promise? What about the promise you made to yourself, to love and respect the person within? When you stop growing spiritually, the person inside ceases to exist. This is nothing to do with religion, it is the essence of mankind. We challenge our minds with all these complicated questions. Building more stress into our day, as if we haven't got enough going on. Do you ever wonder why your neck, shoulders and back are screaming out at you in pain. Make a decision and move on. It's simple, take responsibility and live the life that makes you happy. Why waste time, people will be hurt, but you hurt even more staying in that stale place. These are the constant stories I hear from clients who have done all the above and come to me looking for their answer. I can't and won't tell anyone what to do, I can just listen and offer advice. Ultimately, the key to your happiness lies with you.

THINGS ARE NEVER WHAT THEY SEEM

People sometimes say to me 'I never had any back pain until I started coming here'. Yes, you did you just didn't know it. The problems were already there, but you never felt them. You just felt pain elsewhere in the body. Common areas where you can feel secondary referral pain can be found in your jaw, your arm, down your legs, stomach, and bowel. These all stem from a back that is not working correctly. When a therapist places their hands on your back, healing begins. Tension melts away. People actually fear touch, they do not give themselves permission for their health to be restored. They use every excuse in the book not to get to that appointment; too busy at work, too tired at night to go, too many commitments elsewhere. Valuing yourself allows you to be the happy person you are. When you love and respect yourself, you can then do the same to others. How can you give what you don't know or practice?

Back pain reflects our past, it carries our history and most people who carry a lot of back pain, find it difficult to let go of what happened in the past. Whether it was a difficult childhood, relationship, loss of a loved one, never getting that promotion, missing out on that top job, thinking about it only holds you back in the present. The moment is gone, leave it in the past, learn to move on. Better things are coming your way, you just need to focus on bringing it to you with a positive outlook.

BENEFITS OF MASSAGE

Massage therapy is becoming more widely accepted in the medical community as a credible treatment for many types of back pain and/or as an adjunct to other medical treatments. Research shows that massage therapy has several potential health benefits for back pain sufferers, including:

- Increased blood flow and circulation, which brings needed nutrition to muscles and tissues. This aids in recovery of muscle soreness from physical activity or soft tissue injury (such as muscle strain).
- Decreased tension in the muscles. This muscle relaxation can improve flexibility, reduce pain caused by tight muscles and even improve sleep.
- Increased endorphin levels--the "feel good" chemicals in the brain. This mood enhancer can ease depression and anxiety, which can help reduce pain and speed recovery--particularly important for those suffering from chronic back or neck problems.

Can massage help your back problem? For most of us, the answer is 'yes', since massage is non-invasive and considered very low risk for most people. In addition to physical benefits, certain types of massage have been shown to help psychologically via relaxation and increased production of 'feel good' chemicals that the body naturally produces (endorphins)--helpful for people with both acute back problems and chronic back pain.

LT Therapy was founded through twenty years of research and working with hundreds of clients to develop the winning formula. This enables me to release all forms of muscular neck, shoulder and back pain rapidly with instant results. The advanced technique I developed evolved by pooling together the best massage methods on the market today, then incorporating volcanic heat and ice marble.

PICK & MIX YOUR RECIPE

Key number 1 - Keep active daily

Scientists used to think that strenuous exercise was the only way to improve your health. However, new research suggests that just 30 minutes of moderate physical activity, such as a brisk walk or washing your car, provides most of the health benefits from exercise. The activity doesn't have to be too vigorous. In fact, moderate intensity is best, but even low-intensity activity is better than nothing. While some people may enjoy participating in a regularly scheduled exercise class, others may find it easier to just increase their daily activities. The more vigorous the activity, the more endorphins are released.

The key is to find something that you enjoy doing and do it regularly.

- Go for a brisk walk
- Work in the garden
- Go for a bike ride
- Play golf
- Wash the car
- Walk the dog
- Attend Zumba classes

As you age, you lose muscle and bone mass and may develop problems in your muscles, joints, and bones, so the potential of back pain increases. Regular exercise slows the loss of muscle mass, strengthens bones, and reduces joint and muscle pain. In addition, mobility and balance are improved, which reduces the risk of falling and suffering a serious injury, such as a hip fracture.

It's never too late to start. Physical activity is especially important for older adults, and can help them live independently for as long as possible. A study of frail, wheelchair-bound nursing home residents in their 80s and 90s who participated in a weight lifting program showed marked improvement in their strength and overall functional ability. Staying active also lowers your risk of heart disease or heart attack, lowers blood pressure, controls diabetes and helps you maintain a healthy weight.

TOP TIP TO REMEMBER

On waking every morning before you get out of bed, remember to stretch your body for a few seconds. Watch any animal, especially a cat or dog, before they get up to move, they stretch then move. They are preparing their body for movement without shocking it. If you've been relaxing and sleeping for five hours or more, to suddenly jump out of bed, even if you gently get out of bed, it's like sending a nano tremor through the body. As we lie down, hundreds of times in our lifetime, can you imagine by the time we get to mid-life what these mini jolts are doing to our backs? Wake, Stretch, Move.

KEY NUMBER 2 - DIET

Get detoxing once every three months. Nothing complicated, keep it simple by just cutting out fizzy drinks, alcohol, caffeine, high carbohydrates for seven days, giving the body a chance to re-boot itself. Drink regular filtered water (at least 2.5 litres a day), green tea and herbal tea. It's a great cleansing process. If you are suffering a lot of back pain, incorporate anti-inflammatory foods as follows;

ANTI-INFLAMMATORY FOODS

Fruits and Vegetables - whole fruits, berries, vegetables are all rich in vitamins, minerals, fibre, antioxidants and phytochemicals. Choose green and brightly coloured vegetables and whole fruits such as broccoli, chard, strawberries, blueberries, spinach, carrots and squash. You should eat at least five (and preferably more) servings of fruits and vegetables each day.

Protein Sources - potential anti-inflammatory protein sources include fish and seafood. Oily ocean fish like salmon and tuna is the best because it's high in omega-3 fatty acids. Soy and soy foods such as tofu along with other legumes are the top plant-based protein sources, followed by walnuts, almonds, pecans and Brazil nuts.

Fats and Oils - omega-3 fatty acids are found in cold-water oily fish, flaxseed, and canola oil and pumpkin seeds. Consumption of monounsaturated fatty acids in olive oil, avocados, and nuts has been linked to reduced risk of cardiovascular disease. Other healthful oils include rice bran oil, grape seed oil, and walnut oil.

- Aim for variety.
- Include as much fresh food as possible.
- Minimize your consumption of processed foods and fast food.
- Eat an abundance of fruits and vegetables.

TOP TIP TO REMEMBER

Controlling our stress levels is important as when we are under pressure we crave processed sugary foods. Drink more water and green tea to cleanse your pallet. Take a supplement of Chlorella, a super green food available in tablet or powder. It is a natural algae similar to seaweed but fifty times more powerful. Chlorella has great potential as a supernutrient for the body. Its detoxification abilities make it an important part of a treatment program, especially for those who want to cleanse the body of toxins. Patients with diabetes or fibromyalgia should also consider chlorella, not as a primary treatment, but as part of a program. Hopefully, research will help demonstrate further benefits for heart disease, as chlorella has already proven its benefit in helping to reduce high cholesterol and high blood pressure.

KEY NUMBER 3 - MEDITATION

The meaning of meditation is a practice in which an individual trains the mind or induces a mode of consciousness to release stress.

The term meditation refers to a broad variety of practices that includes techniques designed to promote relaxation, build internal energy or life force, develop compassion, love, patience, generosity and forgiveness. This powerful tool shows you how to take control of your life, that's why it should be practiced twice daily. Create the inner sanctuary that you fail to find on the outside, within you. Make sure you practice when undisturbed. Book time out of your busy schedule to give back to you. You find that when you do, you feel valued, worthy and happy. That in turn radiates out to your partner, children, family, friends, work colleagues and people want to be more like you.

Transcendental Meditation unfolds the full potential of life. Extensive research has found it reduces stress and anxiety resulting in more inner peace, creativity, health, success and happiness. Train, Practice, Master meditation for life. Become a better you.

TOP TIP TO REMEMBER

Don't forget about you. I cannot emphasis this enough. I am harping on about it because you got your back pain in the first place because you did just that, forgot about you. As the song by Simple Minds says, 'Don't you forget about me', that applies to YOU! Take massive action and make that change now. As I said before, it's never too late whatever your age or circumstance, just do it!

KEY NUMBER 4 - TAKE CONTROL

As soon as pain starts in your back and it's beginning to get unbearable, make sure you know what pain killers to take. Whether you are using something natural like breathing control technique, meditation, homeopathy, or pharmaceutical pain killers take control early. This is the key to preventing back pain getting out of control and causing further problems. After five days to seven days, if there is no improvement, get yourself off to the GP for further investigation.

Pain is often mistreated or undertreated and can lead to depression, insomnia, lethargy and reduced physical and mental functioning. Successful control is more likely to be achieved if a proper assessment is made by your doctor, which should include:

- The site of the pain.
- The duration, speed of onset and whether the pain is intermittent or constant.
- The character of the pain - this will indicate whether it is neuropathic or nociceptive.
- Aggravating and relieving factors.
- Impact on daily living.
- Social, emotional and psychological aspects.
- Severity - use of pain scales can make this more objective.

TOP TIP TO REMEMBER

Taking pain killers in a sensible controlled way will not turn you into an addict. Take the right ones suited to your needs and if in doubt check it out. When we are young, we do not feel pain as much and our bodies recover from injury faster. As we age, from 40 plus, recovery takes longer and we feel pain more, so you need to be sensible, not brave or a hero. By taking appropriate painkillers for a short term, you will help your back fully recover, checking with your GP, wherever necessary, on your progress.

My final case study shows that even if you add all the four Keys to your life, fate sometimes has something else in store for you beyond your control.

JOEL'S STORY

Joel formed his Rock Band in the UK in 1994 establishing a large fan base. His band moved to the USA where they became well known for their music, heavily influenced by the likes of David Bowie, Queen and T.Rex. Joel the lead singer and bass guitar player had been my client for almost two years. He came to see me in the UK whenever he was working overseas. He lived in Los Angeles, but came to London to write film scores and work on his own sound.

After twenty years, his band was touring the UK as a thank you to their loyal fans. Joel telephoned me early one Sunday morning to say that he had been on stage in Edinburgh the night before and had slipped whilst playing, hurting his back. He had to be in Manchester on Sunday evening, but couldn't play the way he felt. He asked me if I would be good enough to see him out of clinic hours. I agreed as it was an emergency and rare. If he couldn't play that night, none of the band members could do his main vocal, so the concert would have to be cancelled.

Joel lived a really clean and healthy life out in L.A. He had an amazing diet, didn't touch alcohol, caffeine or red meat. Exercised daily, minimum 30 minutes and meditated twice a day with TM. His back was flexible and in great physical condition. I told him that if there was any inflammation he would have to take control with appropriate pain killers, as I couldn't work on that area.

As I checked his back, I picked up a band of tightness in his mid and lower trapezius, the muscles that lay behind his lungs. Every time he took a breath it hurt. He had already checked himself out in A&E who had confirmed no broken bones, they said it was muscular hence he called me. He needed a fast result in order to get back on stage that night, so who better to call but the Muscle Whisperer. Sometimes my client's can ask the impossible and I will always try to give it to them within reason. I am honest and won't mince my words. He had pulled the muscle right across his back and I would have to work carefully around the area to release it (see Fig 8). Ice marble, then volcanic heat was used to restore the muscle. Sixty minutes later he sat up and took a sharp breath saying 'You're incredible I can breath and it doesn't hurt anymore.'

Joel went on to perform that night and completed the 30 dates on his UK tour without a hitch.

CONCLUSION

Even though the fall was unavoidable, life happens. The reason Joel's back had such a remarkable recovery was because he had such a fantastic work-life balance in place. He had taken my advice when I first met him and made a change for the better. His diet and exercise programme was excellent. He practiced his TM twice a day, even on tour. The natural healing power of the body is simply astounding, if you give it a chance. I manipulated his muscles using LT Rapid Results. Applying the correct technique and manoeuvring toxins away from the area restored total well being and he was able to continue performing.

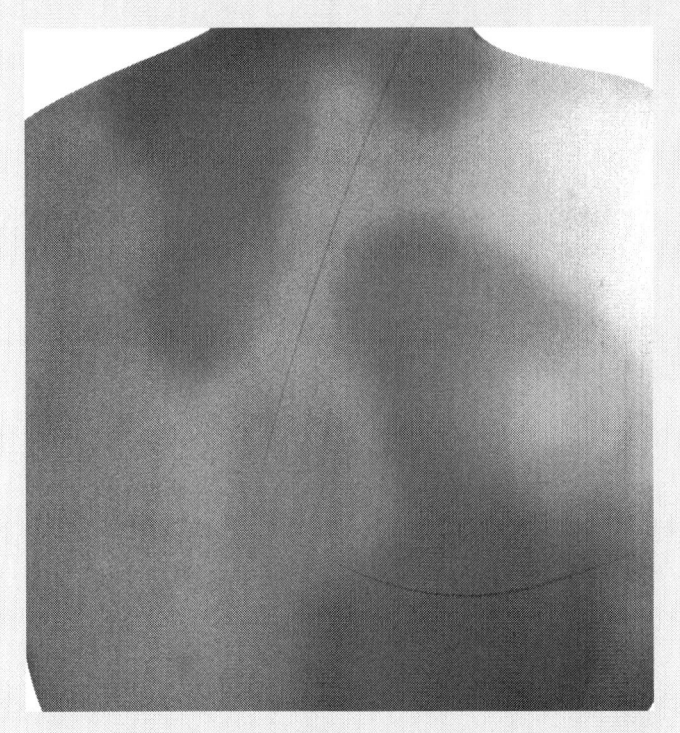

Fig 8 - Photo shows both sides from under shoulder blades to lower back darker emphasising blocked male and female energy.

FINAL WORD

The amazing picture on the front cover of this book, shows chains encasing a back. Each link represents an event or challenging time in our lives, from childhood to present day, that we hold onto deep in our subconscious mind and muscles. The pain is held mainly in our back muscle tissues, as it represents our past, until it is released by 'LT Therapy'. My specialised work as a Muscle Whisperer, enables me to identify and locate key areas that just won't heal with any other treatment. Many clients come to my clinic after they have had various treatments from physiotherapists, chiropractors, sports massage, deep tissue massage, myofascial massage etc, but they still feel that niggling pain in their muscle. I truly commend the work of the technicians of our backs, the physiotherapists, chiropractors, osteopaths, as well as all forms of body massage and energy work, as everyone offers a solution to a person's needs. However, sometimes, a more specialised treatment is required and that's where my work comes in. Reading a person's back muscles is a very specific technique and calls on intuition and a great amount of experience. Knowing when to apply the volcanic heat and ice marble, takes skill and precision, in order to ensure the muscle is treated respectfully, without causing trauma. Focusing on what created the pain originally, means the client feels deep release both mentally and physically, allowing the pain to diminish immediately. It will only return, if the person regularly revisits the event in their mind. It will trigger memory and as muscle has memory, the experience will resurface, causing the acute pain in the back muscle to recur. The links begin to break when we take control of our stress and enforce changes that lead to a better work, life, balance. Daily application is imperative and can be achieved easily, by following the keys as shown in Chapter 8 of this book.

'LT Therapy' is now used as part of a pre and post operative well-being recovery program, for patients who have medical or cosmetic procedures. Private hospitals, clinics and medical groups now ask me to construct for their patients a 'Holistic Well-Being Recovery Programme' as part of their operative package. The idea came about, when a number of people approached me, who were due to have various operations. They found that they were becoming increasingly anxious and worried, prior to the event. By removing and breaking down tight knotty muscles, that had been there, not just because of their apprehension for the impending procedure, but due to previous pressures, their neck, shoulder and back muscles regained immense flexibility. By freeing these muscles, relaxation was restored instantly to mind, body and spirit. Once the consultant had given the client approval for a follow up treatment, after their operation, they would return to me where I applied 'LT Therapy' again, which helped to remove any residual anaesthetic and muscle tightness acquired during the procedure. The client found that their recovery was quicker and their body healed well, due to improved circulation.

Facing daily challenges and fears we have held onto from childhood to present day, will always be reflected somewhere in our back muscles, from neck, shoulders to mid and lower back. No one can ever avoid this, as our thoughts create our physical pain. For many, this concept will be hard to accept, as there will be people adamant that physical pain is ultimately produced from a physical force, but all my clients who I have treated for over twenty years prove otherwise. This book was written to offer you an alternative reason for your back pain and how it was caused, based on the way you reacted to stress. For me, there will always be an emotional reason behind a physical pain. Remember, physical pain is our body's natural warning signal that something is wrong, either due to a physical trauma, such as an accident or it is reacting to an emotional challenge. If you haven't had an accident, then look at what recently challenged you emotionally, then you will understand more about where your neck, shoulder and back pain came from.

If you just learn one thing from this book, then it's been worth writing. I believe knowledge is power and with power comes great responsibility - now where have I heard that line before?

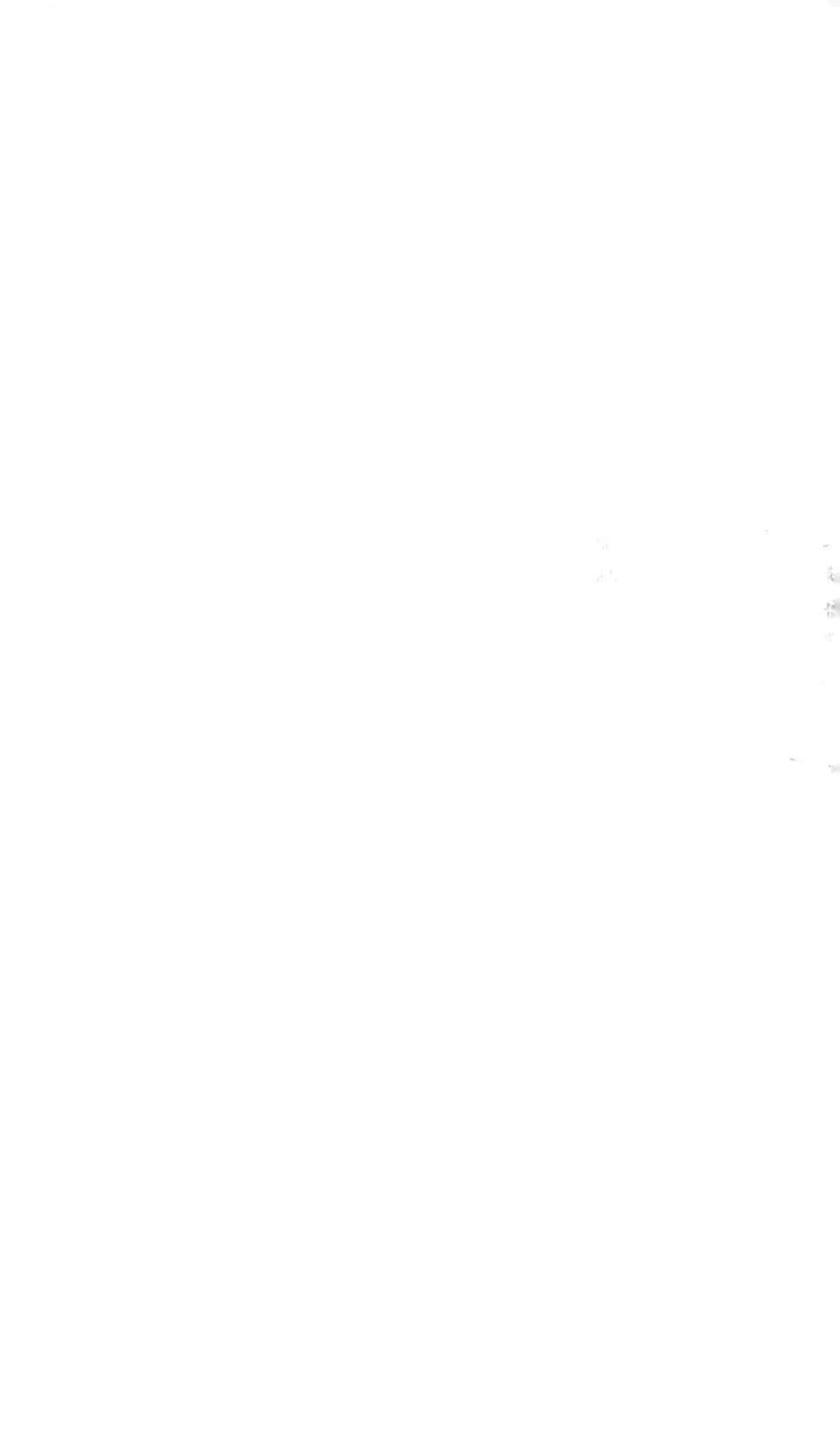

REFERENCES

BOOKS & WEBSITES YOU MAY LIKE TO TRY

Dr Alejandro Junger recommended book:
'Clean: A Revolutionary Program to Restore the Body's natural ability to Heal Itself.'
www.cleanprogram.com

James Duigan recommended book:
'Clean & Lean.'
www.bodyism.com

Dr Norman E. Rosenthal recommended book:
'Transcendence.' Transcendental Meditation
www.tm.org/uk & www.davidlynchfoundation.org.uk

Anthony Robbins recommended book:
'Awaken the Giant Within: How to Take Immediate Control of Your Mental, Emotional, Physical & Financial Life.'
www.tonyrobbins.com

Dr Marilyn Grenville recommended book:
'Fat around the Middle.'
www.marilynglenville.com

Fiona Kirk recommended book:
'2 Weeks in the Fast Lane Diet.'
www.fatbustforever.com

Janey lee Grace recommended book:
'Look Great Naturally.'
www.imperfectlynatural.com

Michael E. Rosenbaum recommended book:
'Chlorella - The sun powered super nutrient and its beneficial properties.'
www.chlorella-europe.com

Albert E. Carter recommended book:
'Rebound Exercise: The Ultimate Exercise for the New Millennium.'

Information on PCD can be found at their website:
www.pcdsupport.org.uk

Bellicon Trampolines available at:
www.ukjuicers.com/BelliconRebounder

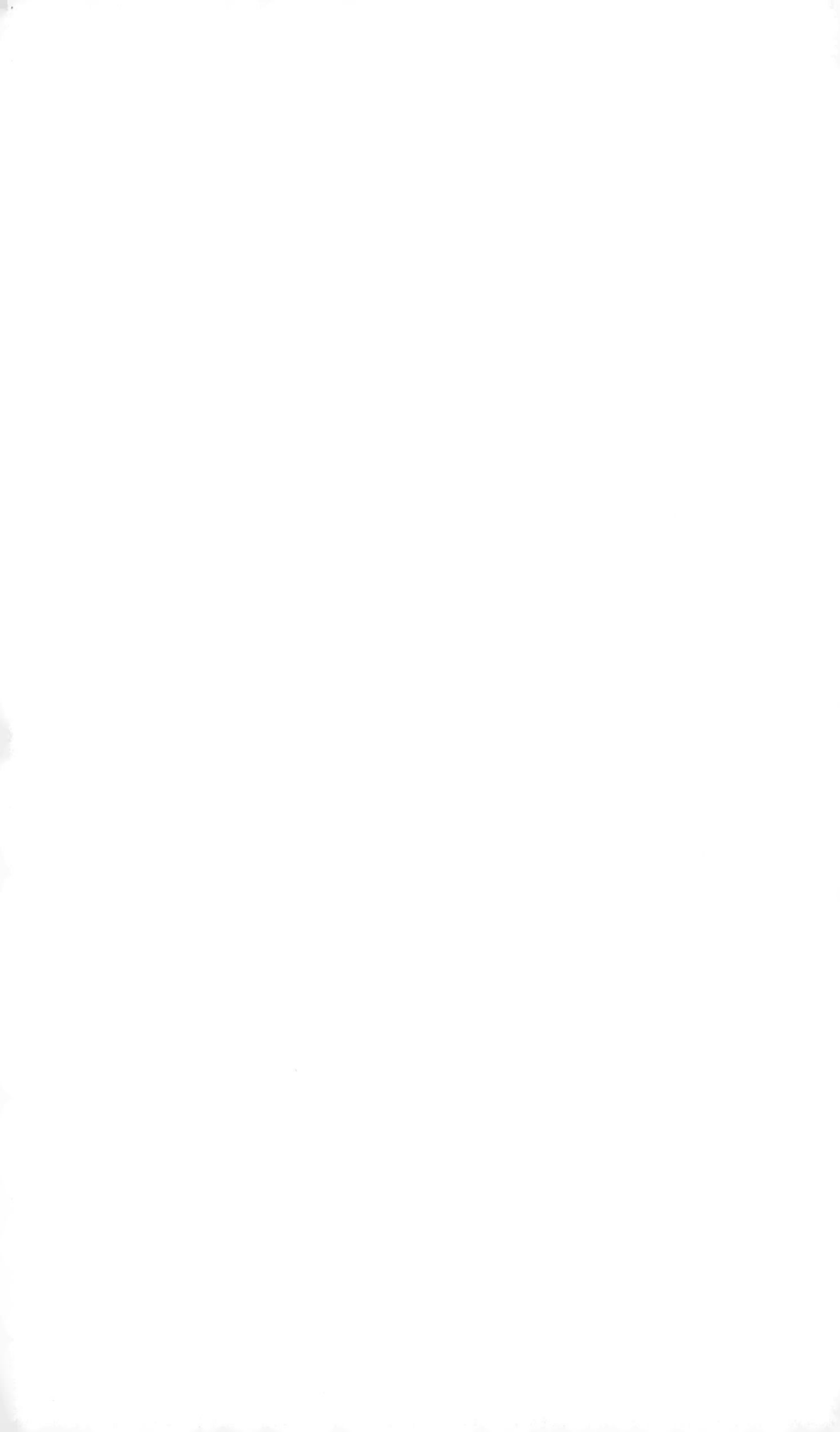

Made in the USA
Charleston, SC
07 October 2014